The **Four** Most Effective Drugless Methods of Deliverance from Insomnia and Universal Method of Drugless Treatment for Depression, Chronic Fatigue Syndrome, other Neurological Diseases and Hypertension

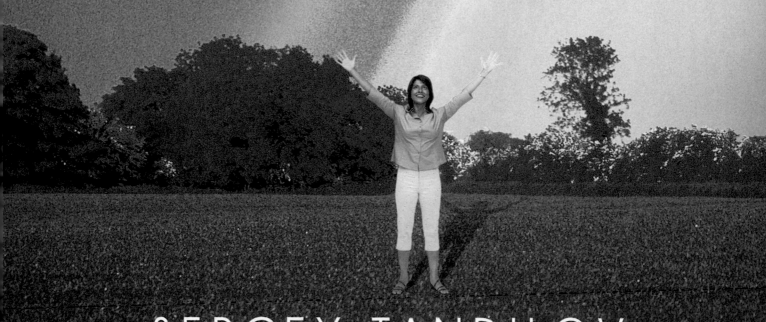

SERGEY TANDILOV

AuthorHouse™ UK Ltd.
1663 Liberty Drive
Bloomington, IN 47403 USA
www.authorhouse.co.uk
Phone: 0800.197.4150

Published by AuthorHouse 03/07/2014

ISBN: 978-1-4918-9424-8 (sc)
*   978-1-4918-9425-5 (e)*

Any people depicted in stock imagery provided by Thinkstock are models,
and such images are being used for illustrative purposes only.
Certain stock imagery © Thinkstock.

This book is printed on acid-free paper.

Because of the dynamic nature of the Internet, any web addresses or links contained in this book may have changed
since publication and may no longer be valid. The views expressed in this work are solely those of the author and do not
necessarily reflect the views of the publisher, and the publisher hereby disclaims any responsibility for them.

authorHOUSE®

The Four Most Effective Drugless Methods of Deliverance from Insomnia and Universal Method of Drugless Treatment for Depression, Chronic Fatigue Syndrome, other Neurological Diseases and Hypertension

SERGEY TANDILOV

CONTENTS

Part 1

The four most effective methods of deliverance from insomnia, three of which permit to manage without soporific

Part 2

Universal method of drugless treatment for depression, chronic fatigue syndrome, other neurological diseases and hypertension

PART 1

The four most effective methods of deliverance from insomnia, three of which permit to manage without soporific

1 General information

More correct from scientific point of view title of the present methods would be **"The four most effective methods of deliverance from initial insomnia, three of which permit to manage without soporific"** since the methods were not tested on those having very serious insomnia, however, it does not belittle significance of the methods, since they permit to get rid of initial insomnia (dyskoimesis or dropping-off to sleep disorder) by special energetic and esoteric ways that seems very humane since all soporifics have side effects, they promote appearance of both physical, and psychological dependences and their ability to provide dream reduces with time since an organism accustoms to the soporifics. Besides, frequent visits to a doctor with an aim to get prescription for new portion of soporific become unnecessary. In a chapter **"7 Additional recommendations for the best dropping-off to sleep"** of the present book, many additional advices are adduced and some of them can be considered as independent methods.

2 Useful information about sleep disturbances

2.1 What are sleep disturbances?

The normal dream necessary for vital activity of the person makes 6-8 hours for adults and 4-6 hours for people of advanced age. Insomnia is characterized by dropping-off to sleep disorder, by disorder of depth and of duration of the dream.

Scientists define several types of sleep disturbances, which declare themselves variously:

1) **Dropping-off to sleep disorders** - the person cannot fall asleep for a long time or he/she does not fall asleep at all. Events and situations of last day as though pass in consciousness, the person tries to find a convenient pose, counts in his head but the dream does not come and process of dropping-off to sleep is stretched for an hour and more;

2) **The superficial dream** - declares itself by feeling of insufficient depth of the dream, frequent night awakenings and difficulties of dropping-off to sleep after them, duration of a night dream is shortened;

3) **Early awakening** – the night dream is short-term, the person wakes up too early. After awakening, there are burdensome feelings, dissatisfaction with the dream, flaccidity, day sleepiness;

4) **Senile insomnia develops at elderly age** - the person falls asleep easily, but quickly wakes up and hardly falls asleep again, the general duration of the dream is shortened. The dream becomes fragmented, superficial, there is a need for a day dream.

There is cognitive information in the Internet about each of these types of sleep disturbances.

Following factors lead to short-term insomnia (from 1 to 3 weeks): Stresses, adaptation disorders, pain syndromes, chronic diseases, receive of stimulant drinks and drugs before going to bed. Elderly people and those who are engaged in brainwork have insomnia especially often.

If insomnia proceeds more than 3 weeks it already is considered chronic. Chronic insomnia often meets at people of elderly and old age.

2.2 Why sleep disturbances are dangerous?

Sleep disturbances can have many sources: These are anxieties, the wrong regimen, too intensive rhythm of life, some illnesses, stresses and psychological traumas. All these disorders lead to that the person feels, in the afternoon, the burdensome sleepiness disturbing him/her to lead habitual way of life.

In the morning, it seems to the person having insomnia that he/she worked all night long. But there is more to come. Sleep disturbances declare themselves in chronic fatigue, dejectedness, inattention and irritability. The constant sleep debt leads to negative changes in appearance, paleness of a skin, shadows under the eyes and also, as it will seem strange, - to formation of excess weight. The organism weakened by a sleep debt cannot any more independently fight even against insignificant disturbances, diseases or infections.

It is possible and it is necessary to struggle with insomnia as it can be at the bottom of many diseases: Of psychological ones, of cardiovascular system (including brain vessels), of diseases of digestive organs. Treatment of a serious form of insomnia represents a difficult task, which it is possible to solve beyond doctor's power only.

2.3 How to restore a normal dream

Now, insomnia is one of the most acute medical problems, which becomes complicated by that there is not such single universal remedy, which would help to everybody as the reasons leading to insomnia are various. Therefore, they use both medical chemical preparations, which it is necessary to take only on the advice of a doctor, and natural remedies.

Chemical preparations, certainly, give fast effect. But quickly - it is not always good. Often, chemical preparations give side effects and cause accustomization. Many people complain of too long influence of drugs leading to the sleepiness in the afternoon and to retardation of thought activity. At taking chemical preparations, there can be a nervous breakdown, concern, reaction retardation, memory weakening, flaccidity. Besides, preparations can cause a headache, dryness in a mouth, nausea, constipations and other more serious abnormalities.

2.4 Insomnia problem at elderly age

The people having senile insomnia should take into consideration that it has chronic character. Remedies against insomnia are prescribed to long term, therefore, threat of their accumulation in the organism increases. Besides, elderly people often have various diseases, which taking the soporific could not be combined with. Therefore, elderly and old people need to choose soporific with special care.

3 The first method of drugless deliverance from dropping-off to sleep disorder

3.1 General recommendations

It is necessary sitting or standing in a bath or shower cabin to mass Sahasrara (cinciput) by shower stream of medium or maximum head (force) imagining that space energy flows into you. Water should be of comfortable temperature, sometimes, it is possible to stimulate yourself with cool or cold water for a short time. It is better to do it before going to bed and it is possible to repeat it in the afternoon too. After shower, sit down in a convenient chair and put on the head a small glass pyramidion or pyramidion made from a stone suitable to your zodiac sign and, through it (pyramidion), send a space stream to Sahasrara (cinciput). Hold the pyramidion on the head 5-10 minutes. The dream will become normalized gradually, in several weeks. Ability of the pyramids and pyramidions to concentrate space energy is known from ancient times and, in this case, curative effect takes place in many respects just thanks to this feature of the pyramids and pyramidions.

3.2 Details

It is necessary to be engaged in the present method one-two weeks and, at the same time, to continue taking the soporific or other drug helping to fall asleep. You should leave off the soporific or other drug helping to fall asleep so: In one-two weeks, it is necessary to start to omit every other day drug intake, i.e. to take drug every other day. You should do so one-one and a half week, and, then, it is possible to stop taking the soporific or other drug helping to fall asleep at all. It is possible also to reduce gradually a dose of the preparation helping to fall asleep.

Experience of people using this method proves that it is possible to be engaged not every day but every other day. It reduces some psychological load caused by occupations by the present method and it is not more difficult to fall asleep than at daily occupations. However, the author of this and other adduced in the present book methods (below, "author") recommends to be engaged every day the first month.

As you already understood, it is necessary to begin each occupation from taking the shower, while which you direct the shower stream of medium or maximum head (force) onto the head and mass Sahasrara (cinciput) imagining that energy of space flows into you. Researches showed that, during the first several minutes after one turns on water flow from a faucet or shower nozzle, water goes polluted and enough harmful at least for internal use. Therefore, the author recommends to turn on water flow from the faucet or shower nozzle on 5 minutes before taking the shower and to take shower after it only. In approximately three weeks after beginning of occupations by the method instead of shower, it is possible, having undressed waist-high and having bent over a washbasin or bath, direct the shower stream of medium or maximum head (force) on the head and to try to exhale in accented way through tense lips and, at exhalations, to imagine that space energy arrives from space into the head and sometimes even into entire body. This procedure can take, at most, 2 minutes. Each 10-15 seconds, it is possible to do a break, i.e. not to direct the stream of the shower onto the head. However, if shower and direction of the shower stream onto the head are unpleasant to you, it is possible to do just wetting the head and to dry it by a towel at once. It is necessary to finish both shower of full value and any kind of wetting the head by cool or cold water (not for long) for pores of your skin would become closed and there would not be uncomfortable feelings next day. As to shower of full value, it is expedient to finish it having directed the stream of cool or cold water not only onto the head but also separately on a trunk, arms and feet. One more recommendation: Try to take shower of full value before occupation with the pyramidion at least once a week. As to an initial period of occupations, the author advises, for the first three weeks, taking just shower of full value instead of wetting the head out of the shower. It is necessary to stand in the shower three-four minutes. Direct the shower stream of medium or maximum head (force) on the head from above and move by the shower nozzle so that a little bit different parts of Sahasrara (cinciput) were processed. In order that the stream of the shower would be the most perceptible it is necessary to do also vertical movements by a hand holding the shower nozzle, i.e. movements in directions up and down. At the same time, exhale through tense lips and inhale through not tense ones. It is better that both exhalations, and inhalations would not be strong, i.e. would be poorly expressed. At each exhalation, imagine that space energy arrives through Sahasrara (cinciput) into the head and sometimes even into entire body. Each 25 seconds do a break. You can just sit approximately 15 seconds. After a shower, there is big sense to dry yourself well and, especially, skin between toes. The matter is that, at the following after the shower occupation with the pyramidion, it is important to be dry and skin between toes and toenails provided that they happen wet every day or every other day can catch a fungus. As to toenails, they should be dried only if they are not affected with the fungus, otherwise, it is possible to extend the fungus carelessly to healthy toes and toenails.

The author advises to be engaged with the pyramidion on the head sometimes in a condition, which its author (certain distinct from the author of the present method person) called "in the key". This condition is reached by a slow raising the arms till they are stretched forward (i.e. the arms should not be directed to the sides) in parallel to the Earth surface and by "listening" to your own sensations and by tuning that the subsequent actions will be carried out in this special condition "in the key". The author recommends not only "listening" to your own sensations but also doing any dictated by intuition movements by the arms, for instance, movements from up to down (holding the arms in front of you) as if repeating movement direction of space energy. It is expedient to do movements by the arms even if you are not in described above in the present paragraph condition "in the key". For increase of efficiency of occupations, it is possible to do movements by the arms above the head as though directing energy of space and palms on the pyramidion and further into the head and sometimes even into entire body. Besides, the author advises to do the accented exhalations through tense lips and, at these exhalations, to imagine that space energy arrives from space through the pyramidion into the head and sometimes even into entire body. As to inhalations at occupation with the pyramidion, it is better to do them through a nose. It is better that both exhalations, and inhalations would not be strong, i.e. would be poorly expressed. Basically, it is possible to be engaged with the pyramidion 5 minutes only but if the method does not give effect, it is necessary to increase time of occupations with the pyramidion up to 10 minutes. If it does not help, it is necessary to be engaged twice a day.

The general duration of each occupation turns out small and, besides, it contains break, which duration is approximately 5 minutes, after which it is necessary to start occupation directly with the pyramidion. It is possible to be engaged either before an hour to going to bed or directly before going to bed. If the method does not give expected effect it is possible to be engaged as well in the afternoon.

The crystal or glass pyramidion with base sides equal to approximately from 4 to 8 centimeters will be suitable for occupations even with the burned by laser in its center zodiac sign image, it is desirable, yours. The pyramidion made from a material (stone) suitable to your zodiac sign with base sides equal to approximately from 4 to 8 centimeters too is even more qualitative from the point of view of effect. Alternation of the crystal or glass pyramidion with the pyramidion made from the material (stone) suitable to your zodiac sign is expedient, i.e., during one occupation, you use one of these pyramidions and during next occupation – the second one etc. There is an opinion that any pyramidion loses its properties in 6 years. Therefore, it is desirable to substitute the pyramidion or pyramidions in 6 years.

While occupation with the pyramidion on the head, it is not necessary to do accented exhalations and described far above in the present subchapter **"3.2 Details"** movements by the arms constantly. It is necessary to do breaks approximately for 15 seconds every minute, i.e. there will be about 4 breaks for these 5 minutes.

The author recommends, at occupations with the pyramidion, to diversify exhalations through tense lips. It is necessary to alternate usual exhalations through tense lips with exhalations through tense lips, thus, as though quietly repeating the English word "flow". It is necessary to have a rest between these types of exhalations for mentioned in the previous paragraph approximately 15 seconds. It seems optimum to the author that each of these types of exhalations lasts for approximately 45 seconds. Sometimes or even always, it is possible to include in one or even in all 45-second cycles of active occupation with the pyramidion both types of exhalations - usual exhalations through tense lips and exhalations through tense lips, thus, as though quietly repeating the English word "flow". Each type of exhalations should last so long how long it is comfortable to you, then, the second type of exhalations should replace it and vise versa. In other words, recommendations can be corrected by you according to your condition and according to that it would be comfortably to you, for example, the cycle can last not 45 seconds but even 20 seconds. Break can last not 15 seconds but 10 seconds. Basically, it is possible to replace or to replace sometimes exhalations through the lips by exhalations through the nose. At all types of exhalations, it is necessary to imagine that space energy flows through the pyramidion and through the top part of the head into the head and sometimes even into entire body. To increase efficiency of occupations, it is possible, while them, to ask mentally the God and your own organism to let you fall asleep easily.

If you have radiculitis, for continuation of occupations with the pyramidion, it is enough to stand all the time at these occupations and you may not move by the arms at all. Just carry out the accented exhalations through tense lips and, at exhalations, and imagine all the same, i.e. imagine that space energy flows through the pyramidion and through the top part of the head into the head and sometimes even into entire body. All the same, effect is the same and you will not provoke radiculitis thus. Even if you have no radiculitis, such mode of occupation with the pyramidion seems to be the most pleasant and the least labor-consuming, at which, about 45 seconds, you stand making exhalations through tense lips, about 15 seconds, you have a rest standing or sitting and, following about 45 seconds, you sit making exhalations through tense lips (it is possible quietly repeating the English word "flow"), then again, have a rest being standing or sitting about 15 seconds etc. In other words, it is better to alternate standing position with sitting one all the time.

3.3 Additional recommendations concerning carrying out the method

It was noticed that the occupation becomes more effective if, before putting the pyramidion on the head, to rub all its facets by two fingers of one of hands.

In case they disconnected hot water or there is no hot water in your house at all, it is possible to boil a pan with water and to mix it, better in enough high basin, with cold water. You should pour such warm water periodically onto your head by some vessel. It is necessary to breathe thus and to imagine the space energy as it is described far above in the present chapter **"3 The first method of drugless deliverance from dropping-off to sleep disorder"**. At the end of procedure, it is necessary to pour cool or cold water on your head couple of times for pores of your skin would become closed and there would not be uncomfortable feelings next day.

As to movements by the arms while occupation with the pyramidion, the author noticed that the tendency inherent in yoga is observed - the higher is the skill of the person being engaged, the less is need of inclusion of dynamic exercises in occupations. Thus, the author's patients started to do reserved movements by the arms recently. However, the latest improvement of the method is combination of movements by the arms from up to down (holding the arms in front of you) as if repeating movement direction of space energy while you are in sitting position and of movements by the arms above the head as though directing energy of space and palms on the pyramidion and further into the head and sometimes even into entire body while you are in standing position. It is possible to do conversely sometimes, i.e. to move the arms from up to down (holding the arms in front of you) while you are in standing position and to move the arms above the head as though directing energy of space and palms on the pyramidion and further in head while you are in sitting position. It is possible not to do long breaks in occupation, thus, since different muscles are involved in these movements by the arms and the arms are not tired. It is possible to do only very small breaks to change sitting position on standing one and vice versa.

One of the author's patients missed one occupation by the present method (he was engaged in the method every other day). The dropping-off to sleep disorder returned to him again. However, it disappeared just after resumption of occupations, which take place every other day at present too. So it is better not to leave off carrying out the method at least after not enough long period of occupations.

3.4 Recommendations concerning pyramidions

Photo of pyramidion:

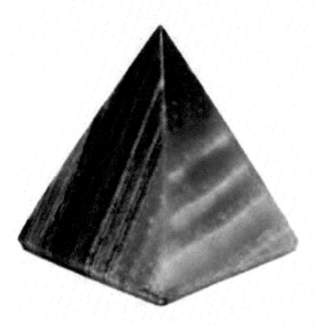

The pyramidion can be bought in a gift shop (shop of gifts) or in small boutique of gifts and souvenirs in majority of shopping centers. Besides, the pyramidion can be bought in majority of online stores of gifts or in majority of Internet auctions.

The author knows exactly that hollow pyramidions, for example, made from a cardboard have the same properties. Somehow, the author made the pyramidion from having mostly gold color box of bonbonniere for an hour. It is necessary to make simple patterns of each facet of the pyramidion with addition of place for joining on glue with other facets of the pyramidion.

The author has two pyramidions - one is made of glass or crystal with sizes 7 cm (i.e. each edge going from a base of the pyramidion to its top has size 7 cm) and 5.8 cm (i.e. each edge of the base of the pyramidion has size of 5.8 cm, i.e. in the base of the pyramidion, there is a square, each side of which has size 5.8 cm); and the second pyramidion made of one of semiprecious stones matching author's zodiac sign with sizes 5.7 cm (i.e. each edge going from the base of the pyramidion to its top has size 5.7 cm) and 5 cm (i.e. each edge of the base of the pyramidion has the size 5 cm, in the base of the pyramidion, there is a square, each side of which has size 5 cm). It is known that the most effective pyramids – pyramids of Mr. Golod have quite extended form, unlike the Egyptian pyramids. Therefore, it is preferable to make the pyramidion of the cardboard with proportions of the bigger pyramidion of the author.

4 The second method of drugless deliverance from dropping-off to sleep disorder

The method described in the present chapter can be applied independently or it can be alternated with occupations with the pyramidion, i.e. one can be engaged in the method described in the given chapter every other day being engaged in occupations with the pyramidion every other day too. For example, be engaged according to the present chapter on Monday and be engaged with the pyramidion on Tuesday and so on. It is possible to be engaged in both methods every day in hard cases of dropping-off to sleep disorder. On the contrary, at mild cases of dropping-off to sleep disorder, it is possible to be engaged every other day, for example, to be engaged according to the given chapter on Monday, not to be engaged on Tuesday at all and to be engaged either according to the present chapter or to be engaged with the pyramidion on Wednesday and so on.

The main gist of this method is that it is necessary to do a salt water compress for the feet for the period of occupations by the method. For this purpose, 2 couples of woolen socks and two cellophane sacks are required. One couple of woolen socks should be wetted in salt warm water, then, it is necessary to dress one sock on each foot and to dress one cellophane sack on each foot over the wet sock. Optimum saturation of water by salt, to be exact, of socks by salt water is reached so: Socks are presoaked in warm water and, then, they are wrung out. Warm water is poured into a soup plate and salt is dissolved in it. It is better to dissolve the mix of a sea salt (3 parts) and rock-salt (1 part). A solution turns out saturated so that not all salt, which volume is half a tea spoon, is dissolved up to the end, however, because socks are wet they aren't saturated with too salt water after their immersion in salt water. After immersion of socks in salt water, it is necessary to wring out them slightly and to put them on feet. Then, it is necessary to put the cellophane sack on each foot. The second couple of woolen socks shouldn't be wetted and it is necessary to dress one of these socks on each foot over cellophane sacks. In order that external socks wouldn't wear out it is possible to sew to each of these socks a sole from a dense material, for example, thin felt. As regards socks wetted in salt water, they should be wetted, after each occupation, in flowing water, wrung out, once again be wetted and wrung out again to get rid of the worked-out salt and, only after that, they should be hung up for drying. By the way, after occupations, it makes big sense to wash out the feet in flowing water too since in the course of these occupations toxic substances, which you shouldn't leave on the skin, are taken away from the skin. Then, it is necessary to dry up the feet and, especially, the skin between toes. As to toenails, they should be dried only if they are not affected with the fungus, otherwise, it is possible to extend the fungus carelessly to healthy toes and toenails.

Occupations have to consist of any simple physical exercises, in breaks between which you should carry out so-called contactless self-massage, i.e. to influence by your palms on your biofield, aura. Information on contactless massage can be found in the Internet. However, in this case, it is a question of the self-massage, which each approach lasts about half-minute. Therefore, it is necessary to be "laconic" and to manage to influence on all parts of your body in these half-minute. Irrespective of whether physical exercises or contactless self-massage are done in the approach, it is necessary to lie after each approach 10-15 seconds.

It is desirable to carry out the method to music or, that is more desirable, to semi-music – the special sounds, which have been recorded on disks for opening chakras. It is recommended to listen to such semi-music via earphones since, only this way, there is the maximum impact on chakras. It is so effective that one of patients of the author achieved that drug helping to fall asleep became not necessary to him even after he ceased to be engaged in the present method (other patients, who listened to music or semi-music during occupations not via earphones, had to be engaged in the present method constantly, i.e. they did not achieve the maximum result). However, he fell asleep without problems. It lasted until scandal with the neighbor happened on the household soil. After that scandal, it became necessary again to start taking drug helping to fall asleep. Conclusion: Avoid scandals and any nervous breakdowns. One of features of occupations of this person was that he did the salt water compress for the feet only during a month (recommended preparatory before listening to disks for opening chakras period) and, then, he did feet bath (salt bath for the feet) about half a year. Approximately in 3 months of occupations with the feet baths (salt baths for the feet), this patient started reducing gradually the dose of soporific and eventually ceased to take this drug. In 1.5 months after refusal of drug intake, the mentioned above patient, who has managed eventually to refuse from drug helping to fall asleep and from occupations by the present method, began to be engaged every other day. In other 1.5 months, he stopped occupations at all. For greater freedom of movements this patient connected earphones to the video recorder via the extender for earphones. These disks can be used also both on the tape recorder (if you got CD disks but not DVD ones) and on the desktop (or the laptop) but it is desirable to use the extender for earphones too.

It makes sense to adduce recommendations concerning the feet bath (salt bath for the feet) from published not by publishing house but by enthusiasts of Sahaja yoga "Methodic textbook for beginners" (on Sahaja yoga; Sahaja yoga is recognized all over the world metascience directed at optimization of opening chakras process): "Before evening meditation, it is good to apply the feet bath (salt bath for the feet) (use water of comfortable temperature, a water level - on an ankle, salt – 1-2 table spoons) within 10 minutes. Then, it is necessary to rinse the feet by pure water, to pour out water from a basin in a toilet and to wash hands. It is very effective technique of removal of negativity through water and earth elements (salt is an earth element)." Recommendations of the author concerning basin, salt and water temperature: It is possible to use both the rock-salt and any sea one. If you use the deep basin (such basins are plastic ones in majority of cases) it is necessary to put into the basin not two spoons of salt as it is told in published not by publishing house but by enthusiasts of Sahaja yoga "Methodic textbook for beginners" (on Sahaja yoga) but four spoons of salt. The author used to put, in the deep basin, three spoons of sea salt with the top (i.e. as much as the spoon is able to contain), one spoon of the rock-salt with the top and mixed water before full dissolution of salt. As regards sea salt, it is usually on sale in drugstores. Salt of ancient sea is preferable. The author liked to provide water temperature in the basin, in the beginning of occupation (before pouring salt), 35-36 degrees Celsius, it is desirable, not more and not less. At the subsequent period of occupation, the author had a desire to reduce water temperature in the basin, in the beginning of occupation (before pouring salt), to 34 degrees Celsius exactly. You should not exceed time of occupation with use of the feet bath (salt bath for the feet) in 30-35 minutes. Mentioned above patient who managed to get rid of need to take drug helping to fall asleep kept the feet in the basin with salt water not constantly. For the period of carrying out the physical exercises mentioned far above in the present chapter and described far below in the given chapter and for the period of so-called contactless self-massage, i.e. influence by one's palms on one's biofield, aura, this person planted himself out of the basin with salt water on a big plastic bag laid on a carpet. It is possible to use waterproof yoga rug instead of the big plastic bag. Then, he took his stand in the basin with salt water again and sat down on the chair. Thus, such element of occupations inherent in occupations with the salt water compress for the feet as short stay in a prone position after each approach irrespective of whether physical exercises or contactless self-massage were carried out was absent thus.

It cannot be excluded that the salt feet baths (salt baths for the feet) have no crucial importance and that the mentioned patient would manage to get rid of need to take drug helping to fall asleep if he did the salt water compresses for the feet instead of the salt feet baths (salt baths for the feet).

It is necessary to make a reservation that, during preparatory before occupations according to the present method period equal to 28 days, this patient listened just to one of the following disks recommended for the preparatory period: CD disk "Antistress" (this disk can be bought, for example, here: [1]), CD disk "Silence temple" (this disk can be bought, for example, here: [2], and it is possible to download it, for example, here: [3]) and CD disk "Healing: on the magic river" (this disk can be bought, for example, here: [4] and it is possible to download it, for example, here: [5]). Just the last disk was used by that patient. Duration of this disk sounding is 50 minutes. Duration of the CD disk "Antistress" is 76 minutes. Author doesn't know about duration of the CD disk "Silence Temple". While listening to the CD disk "Healing: on the magic river", this patient simply lay, however, he started doing the salt water compress for the feet from the first day of the preparatory period.

As regards the disks for opening chakras, they can be bought, for example, having addressed on coordinates (an email sera@san.ru, the ph./fax: +7-(8452)-274-523, mobile ph.: +7-906-152-33-41) adduced on a site [6] in the section "Method of Opening CHAKRAS". The basic thing that can be taken out from this section "Method of Opening CHAKRAS" is that there are three versions of disks for harmonization and possible opening chakras. The first of the said versions are the CD disks made by pioneer of this possibility of harmonization and opening chakras by means of sounds – U.S. Company "FOTON ENTERPRISES, LTD". These disks contain only record of sounds and, as the author knows, they are the most expensive. One more characteristic of these disks is that they are produced individually for each customer provided that this person knows date of his/her birth with an accuracy of an hour and knows the time zone of a place of his/her birth. And one more characteristic – these disks are with the shortest duration of sounding – about 20 minutes. These disks are described on the Internet page [1]. The second of the mentioned above in the present paragraph versions of disks are the DVD disks made in Russia and not by the individual order, they are identical to everybody. These disks contain both record of sounds and record of abstract changing images. These disks are the cheapest. They are described on the Internet page [7]. One more characteristic of these disks – duration of their sounding varies from 29 to 35 minutes depending on each concrete disk. The third of the mentioned above in the present paragraph versions of disks are the DVD disks made in Russia by the individual order. It also as well as in case of the American disks means that the customer has to know date of his/her birth with an accuracy of an hour and to know the time zone of a place of his/her birth. These disks are described on the Internet page [8].

The effect from listening to the second version of the disks appears not so quickly, unlike effect from listening to the disks of the first and third versions. However, the disks of the second version can be used by everybody, while, the disks of the first and third versions can be used by the person, by whose date of birth and time of day of birth they are made. If these disks are used by some other person they can bring harm to this person.

If there is a need to cut down expenses, please, take into consideration that it is not recommended to buy less than four different disks on harmonization of chakras. There are 7 chakras in the human organism and there is a separate disk for activation of each chakra, i.e. there are 7 disks concerning chakras themselves in all. There is an opinion that process of harmonization of chakras is similar to erection of building. They start to build beginning from the ground floor till the last one. Therefore, it is desirable to buy disks on harmonization of at least following bottom chakras: Muladhara, Svadhistana, Manipura and Anahata. As to such recommendations adduced in methodic textbook to each disk for harmonization of any chakra as various mental imaginations, they are actual only in case of use of these disks according to their destination but not for treatment of dropping-off to sleep disorder.

Besides, as it was mentioned above, there must be one disk intended for preparatory period, for instance, CD disk "Antistress" and there must be one CD disk intended for balanced condition training on all chakras, which (CD disk) is named "Balancing of all chakras". All these disks can be bought if to apply to representatives of the site [6], for instance, on their email sera@san.ru. As regards CD disk "Antistress" or other similar disks for preparatory period, they can not be bought if you do not hope to get rid of necessity to take drug helping to fall asleep. However, if you want to manage without drug helping to fall asleep it is better to buy CD disk "Antistress" or other similar disk for preparatory period and to provide, for yourself, the preparatory period. Please, take into consideration that payment to representatives of the site [6] can be done by electronic payment system PayPal.

Taking into consideration that, at occupations by this method, it is necessary to make various movements, wireless earphones seem the most convenient, however, principle of their work – receiving a radio signal – can lead, at some supersensitive (to a radio signal) people, to that dropping-off to sleep disorder can be aggravated. However, such supersensitivity is rare. As regards movements at occupations by this method, rotations by the arms or rotations by the arms with the dumbbells clamped in them, knee-bends, smooth movements, characteristic to such disciplines as Chi gung (Qigong) and Wushu, exercise for a press (from a prone position on a back to raise a torso and to try to reach by the hands to the feet) seem optimum. At rotations by the arms, the right arm rotates in a humeral joint clockwise, and the left one – in opposite to clockwise direction. It is enough to make 10 rotations but if it isn't difficult, make more rotations, up to 25 ones. At rotations by the arms with the dumbbells clamped in them, both arms start carrying out rotary motions similar to those when carrying out described above in the present paragraph rotations by the arms without dumbbells. In the beginning, synchronous rotations by the arms with dumbbells in the following directions are carried out too: The right arm rotates clockwise, and left one – in opposite to clockwise direction. Thus, elbow joints in different arm positions are bent at different value. It is caused by that, at rotating dumbbells at the same time both in front of yourself and a little sideways from yourself, it is necessary to provide a condition of as much as possible long being of dumbbells in the maximum proximity from each other when they almost meet near the bottom of your stomach and reach level of top of your breast. Thus, it is necessary to concentrate on development of the internal energy, which, by the way, provides keeping such trajectory of dumbbells. Rotations of the arms with dumbbells are to be in quantity not more than 12. Anyway, it seems optimum to allow for each approach with any type of movements not more time than each approach with contactless self-massage takes, i.e. not more than half-minute. As for the general duration of occupations with the salt water compress for the feet, they have to last approximately 15-35 minutes each. If before the end of occupation, the salt water compress for the feet described far above in the present chapter **"4 The second method of drugless deliverance from dropping-off to sleep disorder"** seems to you too cold it is necessary to interrupt occupation having removed the salt water compress and having wiped the feet by a towel. Then, it is necessary to be engaged already without the salt water compress. Upon the termination of occupation, it is necessary to wash the feet by flowing warm water and to wipe them dry including places between toes as it is described in a subchapter **"3.2 Details"** of the present book.

5 The third method of deliverance from dropping-off to sleep disorder

The method described in the present chapter can be applied independently or it can be alternated every other day with occupations with the pyramidion or with occupations with the salt water compress for the feet. For example, be engaged according to this chapter on Monday, while, be engaged with the pyramidion on Tuesday and on Wednesday - with the salt water compress for the feet, etc. It is possible to be engaged in two or three methods every day in hard cases of dropping-off to sleep disorder. On the contrary, at mild cases of dropping-off to sleep disorder, it is possible to be engaged every other day, for example, to be engaged according to the present chapter on Monday, not to be engaged on Tuesday at all and to be engaged either according to the given chapter or to be engaged with the pyramidion or with the salt water compress for the feet on Wednesday and so on.

The main essence of this method is that it is necessary to do a body wrapping on the basis of 8-10% solution of alimentary salt. It is better to use the rock-salt since other types of salt contain an alimentary additive, which is undesirable to the organism, especially taking into consideration that 100 grams of salt is spent on each procedure. Two couples of cotton linen, each of which should represent an undershirt with long sleeves and underpants, will be necessary for the body wrapping. 100 grams of salt should be dissolved in 1 liter of warm or very warm water. It is desirable to open a tap before gathering this liter of water and to allow leaking to water 5 minutes since it is known that water with harmful impurity goes out of the tap the first 5 minutes. One couple of linen is doused in prepared by you 8-10% solution of the rock-salt (see above in the present paragraph) and is put on a naked body, which is also desirable for moistening previously in the same 8-10% solution of the rock-salt salt. The second dry couple of linen is put on over the first moist one. The usual house clothes or if it is cool also a woolen jumper and additional pair of house trousers are put on over. It is desirable to do this procedure not less than 3 hours. If you decide to do its larger quantity of time, check whether the linen is too dried up. If the linen is dried up too much, it is necessary to take off everything, to douse the first couple of linen in new 8-10% solution of the rock-salt salt prepared in the same way and again to put on everything. This is rather effective procedure and its duration should be led up to maximum gradually beginning from 3 hours. However, usually it is enough to carry out this procedure during 3-5 maximum 6 hours a day.

If during the first procedure of the body wrapping you feel that your genitourinary organs run cold, take off house trousers and both underpants, one of which were doused by you in 8-10% solution of the rock-salt and, before putting them on again, put on several pants, one of which can be woolen. After the end of procedure of the body wrapping or just before going to bed or in an interval between the end of procedure of the body wrapping and going to bed, it is desirable to take shower to wash away the salt remains from the skin. If not to make it it becomes difficult to fall asleep.

It is desirable to rinse, right after the end of each procedure of the body wrapping, just both pairs of linen, which were used for these procedures but not just that pair of linen, which you doused in salt water, and to hang them out to dry and be ready for your following occupation planned on the next day.

Everything is individually at such procedures, however, experience shows that, in majority of cases, if to do the body wrapping a month for 6 hours a day, after gradual decrease of duration of these procedures and the subsequent full termination of their carrying out, it is possible to get rid of the exacerbation of dropping-off to sleep disorder preceding the beginning of carrying out these procedures. Sometimes, it is enough to do the body wrapping 15 days 5 hours a day to get rid of the exacerbation of dropping-off to sleep disorder. However, at present, there is no experience yet of refusal from the drugs helping to fall asleep thanks to the described body wrapping.

It is important to reduce time of carrying out procedures of the body wrapping gradually, approximately, for an hour a day. After achievement of time of carrying out this procedure 1 hour, the next day, carry out the procedure during half an hour and, the next day, do not carry out this procedure but replace it by one occupation according to the previous chapter **"4 The second method of drugless deliverance from dropping-off to sleep disorder"** of the present book (with the salt water compress for the feet or feet bath (salt bath for the feet)). Next day, it is possible not to do any of these procedures. If not to act in this way and to stop occupations by the body wrapping right away, on the contrary, it is possible to earn an insomnia exacerbation, which will last several days. Therefore, if even you carry out wrapping every other day instead of every day, reduce time of carrying out these procedures also gradually.

For intensifying effect of the method of deliverance from dropping-off to sleep disorder described in the previous chapter **"4 The second method of drugless deliverance from dropping-off to sleep disorder"** of the present book, it is possible, instead of the salt water compress for the feet or, probably, instead of feet bath (salt bath for the feet), to do the body wrapping described in the present chapter. All the rest (movements and contactless self-massage) should be carried out according to the previous chapter **"4 The second method of drugless deliverance from dropping-off to sleep disorder"** of the present book. For even larger intensifying effect of the method of deliverance from dropping-off to sleep disorder it is possible to combine a way described in the previous chapter **"4 The second method of drugless deliverance from dropping-off to sleep disorder"** of the present book and in the present chapter, i.e. having executed the body wrapping and having been occupied according to the previous chapter **"4 The second method of drugless deliverance from dropping-off to sleep disorder"** of the present book, it isn't necessary to take off anything that makes the body wrapping and it is necessary to sustain the body wrapping the necessary time.

If you have a weak heart, the author doesn't recommend doing the body wrapping more than 15 days not more than 5 hours a day and only once in life. If even you have a healthy heart, the author doesn't recommend doing the body wrapping more than a month not more than 6 hours a day and only once in life too.

6 The fourth optional method of drugless deliverance from dropping-off to sleep disorder

Generally speaking, the presented method is universal. It helps from many problems. I recommend to type in any Search Engine key phrase "EFT tapping pdf". EFT means Emotional Freedom Technique. At least one document in PDF format describing the method will be available. As regards insomnia, I recommend to type in any Internet Search Engine key phrase "EFT tapping insomnia". At least one Internet page [9] with different demonstration videos will be available. The main video of this Internet page is not the most important. The matter is that videos concerning EFT tapping against insomnia are intended for different reasons why insomnia appeared. For instance, the main video of the Internet page [9] is intended for cases when insomnia is caused by inability to relax enough to fall asleep. As regards video titled "4 Simple Steps to Blissful Sleep", it is intended for cases when insomnia is caused by stress. As far as video titled "EFT Yourself to Sleep (Emotional Freedom Technique)" is concerned, it is intended, for instance, for cases when insomnia is caused by the fact that a person trying to fall asleep is afraid of that the night will be sleepless. Links of these videos are not adduced in the present book since they can be found by search using their titles "4 Simple Steps to Blissful Sleep" and "EFT Yourself to Sleep (Emotional Freedom Technique)" on the Internet page [9] and on video-sharing website [10].

If the Internet page [9] becomes inaccessible you can try to open another Internet page representing one of pages of video-sharing website [10] with the main video of the Internet page [9]. Thus, this direct link is following: [11]. Other, not main videos from the Internet page [9] and other videos concerning this subject as well are presented in the Internet on video-sharing website [10] too. Their clickable icons are adduced on the right side of the Internet page [11]. There are videos among them, which do not represent EFT (Emotional Freedom Technique). One of such videos titled "3 Exercises to Overcome Insomnia, Stop Thinking so Much and Get a Good Night's Sleep" is intended for those whom too many thoughts visit when they go to bed. Link of this video is not adduced in the present book since this video can be found by search using its title "3 Exercises to Overcome Insomnia, Stop Thinking so Much and Get a Good Night's Sleep" on the Internet page [9] and on video-sharing website [10].

Hard cases of insomnia and dropping-off to sleep disorder need more time of occupations than several days, which it is said in the mentioned above in the previous paragraphs of the present chapter main video of the Internet page [9] about. Thus, another English-language video, which link of its Russian translation only is known to the author, informs that 3 months of occupations by EFT tapping against insomnia were necessary for a woman with hard case of insomnia to get rid of it. It is said also about this woman that she carried out EFT tapping against insomnia several times a day, while, it is recommended in the main video of the Internet page [9] to carry out EFT tapping against insomnia once a day before going to bed. Author's experience says that it is not enough to carry out EFT tapping against insomnia once a day only and it is not enough to carry out EFT tapping against insomnia several days only. It is necessary to carry out EFT tapping against insomnia approximately 5 times a day during at least 3 months. However, if you have already begun to take drug helping to fall asleep it's unlikely that you will be able to get rid of necessity to take this drug. Thus, EFT tapping against insomnia is drugless on condition that you did not begin to take drug helping to fall asleep. However, as it follows from one of documents in PDF format available in the Internet and describing EFT tapping one person who suffered from insomnia and who took soporific recovered by the EFT method aimed on levelling of psychological reasons for his illness and, under observation of the doctor, he ceased to take soporific.

Following phrases are used for EFT tapping against insomnia shown in the main video of the Internet page [9]: "Even though I find it hard to fall asleep, I choose to relax and sleep easily", "Find it hard to fall asleep", "Can't get asleep at night", "Can't fall asleep", "I choose to relax and sleep easily", "I choose to fall asleep easily", "I choose to relax and fall asleep easily", "I choose to relax and sleep easily", "I can't fall asleep" and "I find it hard to fall asleep". EFT tapping against insomnia shown in the main video of the Internet page [9] distinguishes by the fact that it is necessary to carry out 3 repetitions of cycles of the tapping (precisely, cycles of the tapping while pronouncing phrases next to the first one - "Even though I find it hard to fall asleep, I choose to relax and sleep easily"; tapping on top of Head point is carried out in the very end once only) successively and by the fact that it is recommended to carry out, after the third cycle, tapping on usually non-obligatory point - Top of Head one. As regards the first phrase "Even though I find it hard to fall asleep, I choose to relax and sleep easily", it is necessary to pronounce it when tapping on so called karate chop point, which exists on each palm and it does not matter which palm you choose as it follows from one of videos concerning EFT tapping against insomnia. It is necessary to adduce information about which phrase is pronounced while tapping on this or that point (it is necessary to tap 5-9 times on each point besides karate chop point, which it is necessary to tap on all the time you pronounce the first phrase "Even though I find it hard to fall asleep, I choose to relax and sleep easily" 3 times):

Tapping on the first point:

Karate chop point - "Even though I find it hard to fall asleep, I choose to relax and sleep easily"

The first cycle of tapping:

Eyebrow point - "Find it hard to fall asleep"

Side of Eye point - "Find it hard to fall asleep"

Under Eye point - "Can't get asleep at night"

Under Nose point - "Find it hard to fall asleep"

Chin point - "Find it hard to fall asleep"

Collarbone point - "Can't get asleep at night"

Under Arm point - "Can't fall asleep"

The second cycle of tapping:

Eyebrow point - "I choose to relax and sleep easily"

Side of Eye point - "I choose to relax and sleep easily"

Under Eye point - "I choose to fall asleep easily"

Under Nose point - "I choose to relax and fall asleep easily"

Chin point - "I choose to relax and sleep easily"

Collarbone point - "I choose to relax and fall asleep easily"

Under Arm point - "I choose to relax and fall asleep easily"

The third cycle of tapping:

Eyebrow point - "Can't fall asleep"

Side of Eye point - "I choose to relax and sleep easily"

Under Eye point - "I find it hard to fall asleep"

Under Nose point - "I choose to relax and sleep easily"

Chin point - "I can't fall asleep"

Collarbone point - "I choose to fall asleep easily"

Under Arm point – "I can't fall asleep"

Tapping on the last point:

Top of Head point - "I choose to relax and fall asleep easily"

Then, inhale deeply, relax and exhale.

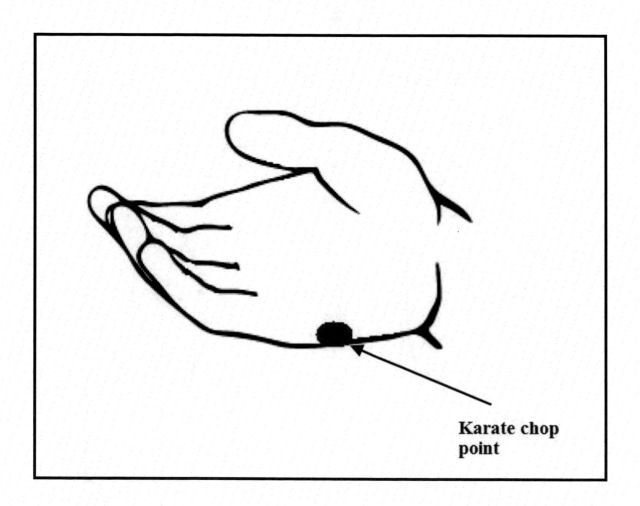

**Karate chop
point**

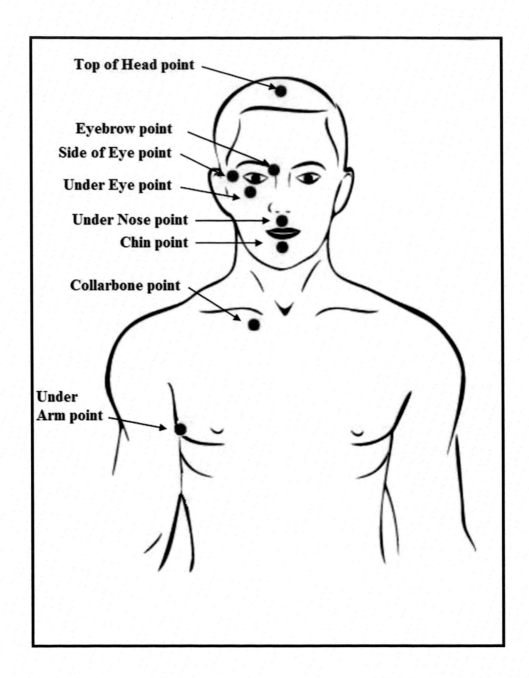

Please, pay attention that as it follows from video presented on the Internet pages [9] and [11], collarbone point represents, in fact, several points.

Author advises to improve EFT tapping against insomnia by addition of several else points on opposite side of your body. By the way, it follows from at least one video concerning EFT tapping against insomnia available on video-sharing website [10] that it is possible to tap on these additional points. Thus, improved version EFT tapping against insomnia will have following view:

Tapping on the first point:

Karate chop point - "Even though I find it hard to fall asleep, I choose to relax and sleep easily"

The first cycle of tapping:

Eyebrow point - "Find it hard to fall asleep"

Side of Eye point - "Find it hard to fall asleep"

Side of another Eye point - "Find it hard to fall asleep"

Under Eye point - "Can't get asleep at night"

Under another Eye point - "Can't get asleep at night"

Under Nose point - "Find it hard to fall asleep"

Chin point - "Find it hard to fall asleep"

Collarbone point - "Can't get asleep at night"

Under Arm point - "Can't fall asleep"

Under another Arm point - "Can't fall asleep"

The second cycle of tapping:

Eyebrow point - "I choose to relax and sleep easily"

Side of Eye point - "I choose to relax and sleep easily"

Side of another Eye point - "I choose to relax and sleep easily"

Under Eye point - "I choose to fall asleep easily"

Under another Eye point - "I choose to fall asleep easily"

Under Nose point - "I choose to relax and fall asleep easily"

Chin point - "I choose to relax and sleep easily"

Collarbone point - "I choose to relax and fall asleep easily"

Under Arm point - "I choose to relax and fall asleep easily"

Under another Arm point - "I choose to relax and fall asleep easily"

The third cycle of tapping:

Eyebrow point - "Can't fall asleep"

Side of Eye point - "I choose to relax and sleep easily"

Side of another Eye point - "I choose to relax and sleep easily"

Under Eye point - "I find it hard to fall asleep"

Under another Eye point - "I find it hard to fall asleep"

Under Nose point - "I choose to relax and sleep easily"

Chin point - "I can't fall asleep"

Collarbone point - "I choose to fall asleep easily"

Under Arm point – "I can't fall asleep"

Under another Arm point – "I can't fall asleep"

Tapping on the last point:

Top of Head point - "I choose to relax and fall asleep easily"

Then, inhale deeply, relax and exhale.

7 Additional recommendations for the best dropping-off to sleep

It is recommended for the best dropping-off to sleep:

1. Not to watch TV;

2. To air a bedroom;

3. To make walk;

4. To drink the drops of a so-called somnolent mixture dissolved in water. This admixture represents a mixture of Corvalolum and tinctures of motherwort (leonurus), hawthorn, peony and valerian roots. You should mix with a small amount of water (approximately 25 ml) so many drops of sleepy mixture how old you are. Not to cause accustomization to this somnolent admixture, it is possible to pass, for a week or two weeks, to taking the medication having a natural origin, New-Passitum after month of taking the somnolent admixture. New-Passitum is tasty medication and, therefore, its form in the form of liquid is preferable. It seems optimum to drink the drops of so-called somnolent mixture dissolved in water or New-Passitum approximately 40 minutes before going to bed;

5. To eat a small portion of food. The small portion of food can be, for example, crisp bread ring and/or bread crisp and/or piece of bread and, maybe, not big part of some vegetable. It seems optimum to eat such small portion of food approximately 20 minutes before going to bed;

6. To take shower;

7. To take comfortable pose in a warm bed (if is necessary to use a hot-water bag);

8. To sleep on an abdomen without a pillow. It is desirable to lie previously approximately half a minute on one's right side at first and, then, to lie approximately half a minute on one's left side. If it doesn't help, it is necessary to add lying on the back too approximately for a minute. It is desirable to sleep on the firm surface. The author sleeps on a folded twice woolen thin (non-stuffed) blanket laid on wooden boards. Use natural boards instead of a particle board, which is cancerogenic;

9. Recommendation demanding discussion with a doctor: For falling asleep, taking such antidepressants as, for instance Ziprexa, Olanzapine or Zalasta approximately for an hour before going to bed helps well. These preparations have the same active ingredient and, unlike soporifics, they have minimum side effects. These preparations can be bought without the prescription too. It is necessary to use search in the Internet for this purpose it is better having tried different key phrases (for instance, "to buy Zalasta") and different Search Engines. However, there is an opinion that the drugs purchased without the prescription, are insufficiently refined. Any drug against insomnia works twice more effectively if to divide it

on 2 equal parts and to drink them one after another with a break 10-15 minutes. It is possible to divide drug on 3 and even 4 equal parts and to drink them one after another with a break 5 minutes or 4 minutes, accordingly, that is still more effective. It is known that Ziprexa, Olanzapine and Zalasta do not cause accustomization. However, just in case, it is possible to take, instead of them, a small dose (for instance, 25 mg) of Azaleptinum or Clozapine (Clozapinum) one time in three days. Though, it is better to take only Azaleptinum or Clozapine (Clozapinum) in that case only if Ziprexa or Olanzapine either Zalasta seem to you excessively expensive. Azaleptinum and Clozapine (Clozapinum) also can be bought without prescription with use of the Internet. The author noticed such pattern: If any of his patients was not able to fall asleep all night long, for the next evening, patient's usual dose of Ziprexa or Olanzapine either Zalasta or Azaleptinum either Clozapine (Clozapinum) was insufficient for falling asleep. There are two exits: To raise slightly dose of Ziprexa or Olanzapine either Zalasta or Azaleptinum either Clozapine (Clozapinum) or soon after going to bed in the absence of possibility to fall asleep to take warm shower, which should be finished by short-term cool or cold shower. Usually, it helps to fall asleep without need to enlarge dose of Ziprexa or Olanzapine either Zalasta or Azaleptinum either Clozapine (Clozapinum) and, therefore, it seems preferable. Often several next nights or many next nights, it is necessary to take such shower to fall asleep. However, it is better than to enlarge dose of Ziprexa or Olanzapine either Zalasta or Azaleptinum either Clozapine (Clozapinum). It is possible to exclude need to take the shower at night if to wake up and get up at least on half an hour earlier than usually. Certainly, it is necessary to try that any of nights would not be completely sleepless. The same warm shower, which should be finished by short-term cool or cold shower, will help to cope with it. It is appropriate here to remind information adduced far above in a subchapter **"3.3 Additional recommendations concerning carrying out the method"** of the present book: "In case they disconnected hot water or there is no hot water in your house at all, it is possible to boil a pan with water and to mix it, better in enough high basin, with cold water. You should pour such warm water periodically onto your head by some vessel… At the end of procedure, it is necessary to pour cool or cold water on your head couple of times for pores of your skin would become closed and there would not be uncomfortable feelings next day." If the shower does not help, it is necessary to take additional dose of Ziprexa or Olanzapine either Zalasta or Azaleptinum either Clozapine (Clozapinum), for instance, the same 25 mg or even 12.5 mg of Azaleptinum or Clozapine (Clozapinum). Such additional dose taken after going to bed and after shower will have influence neither towards augmentation nor towards decrease on the dose of Ziprexa or Olanzapine either Zalasta or Azaleptinum either Clozapine (Clozapinum) habitual for your organism. It is better to divide a tablet of any drug by a sharp knife. The knife should be ground before each division of the tablet. It allows dividing the tablet almost into equal parts, whereas not ground knife divides the tablet not into equal parts. Dividing of the tablet will be still more precise if to make it on a wide plate but not on some plastic cutting board. If nevertheless, it did not turn out to divide the tablet into equal parts you can cut off a small piece from the biggest part of the parted tablet and take it (the small piece) with smaller part of the parted tablet;

10. Recommendation, which can suit not to everybody: Before going to bed, it is necessary to drink 2 glasses of water having washed down with them a salt pinch. It must be kept in mind that a large amount of salt can make water as much harmful for health as sea water is.

11. Scientists of Medical School of Pittsburgh University found out that when those suffering by insomnia put on cooling hat for the night they slept not less strong than those who have no problems with dream. For now, while, cooling hats aren't present on sale try the strategy offered by doctor Lawrence Epstein, the medical director of the Dream Center in Brighton, the State of Massachusetts: To reduce body temperature (and the brain temperature!) take a warm bath for half an hour-hour before going to bed. In reply, the body will start own cooling system. Air temperature in a bedroom has to be not more than 18 °C.

12. If one suffering from dropping-off to sleep disorder goes to bed at the same time each day it makes it easier to fall asleep. If you decide to adhere to this advice try to go to bed approximately at the same time and turn out light in the room always at the same time accurate within a second. Absolutely exact clock or watch are a big rarity and, therefore, buy any clock or watch with indication of seconds on the liquid crystal dial and expose exact time on them every day being guided by signals of exact time by radio or television.

13. If to change time of going to bed on approximately two minutes later than usually it facilitates a task to fall asleep. However, such disadvantage is in this tactics that, eventually, you will displace time of going to bed very considerably towards later time. Therefore, resort to this tactics seldom.

14. Physical activity carried out at any time of day makes it easier to fall asleep. Stroll on a bicycle or occupation on an exercise bicycle help in perfect way. Stroll on the bicycle can last, for example, 15 minutes to half an hour a day. Occupation on the exercise bicycle can last, for example, 15 minutes. Try to be engaged every day since organism gets accustomed to physical activity and absence of the latter in some day leads to inability to fall asleep. If you have to miss stroll on the bicycle or occupation on the exercise bicycle, in this day, you can be engaged according to the chapter **"4 The second method of drugless deliverance from dropping-off to sleep disorder"** of the present book and you will fall asleep nevertheless. If even you have to leave off physical activity at all you can be once engaged according to the chapter **"4 The second method of drugless deliverance from dropping-off to sleep disorder"** of the present book instead of physical activity and all the next days can include neither physical activity nor occupation according to the chapter **"4 The second method of drugless deliverance from dropping-off to sleep disorder"** of the present book, i.e. you can leave off physical activity at all without exacerbation of insomnia.

15. There are hypnotizers who cure insomnia and dropping-off to sleep disorder by hypnosis. The hypnotizers can be found by search in the Internet.

8 Application of the method in case of total absence of dream

It is possible to assume that in those exceptional cases when the patient completely has no dream even at intake of drug helping to fall asleep, ability to fall asleep will be restored at occupations with the pyramidion and, at adding occupations with the salt water compress for the feet, it will become possible to fall asleep without drugs. It cannot be excluded that despite daily occupations both with the pyramidion and with the salt water compress for the feet, it will become possible to fall asleep only on condition of taking drug helping to fall asleep. In very hard cases, it is possible to follow also to the advices given in the previous chapter **"7 Additional recommendations for the best dropping-off to sleep"** of the present book.

9 Testimonials of the persons using the method

"I am so happy to manage without drugs and, trust me, it is difficult and troublesome to obtain them that these summary 15 minutes when I take shower or wet the head and, then, sit and stand with the pyramidion on the head each alternate day and when I am occupied with the salt water compress for the feet for half an hour sometimes seem to me as somewhat unrealistically good."

"This method makes it possible to grope ways of recovery and to recover from insomnia, which is considered very difficult to treat."

PART 2

Universal method of drugless treatment for depression, chronic fatigue syndrome, other neurological diseases and hypertension

1 Introduction

Working speaking for itself title of this method was "Methods of active self-regulation for deliverance from depression, chronic fatigue syndrome and hypertension (Method of magic phrases and movements)".

Begin with reading a chapter **"2 General information"** of the present book. Then, see a demonstration video, link of which is adduced in a chapter **"Bibliography"** of the given book (see source of information [12]). After that, read a chapter **"6 The text of the author of the method pronounced by him in a demonstration video"** of the present book, then, read a chapter **"8 Notes"** of the given book. After that, read chapters **"3 Part one of the universal method of drugless treatment for depression, chronic fatigue syndrome, other neurological diseases and hypertension"** and **"4 Keys to the method"** of the present book.

Basically, you can not do feet bath (salt bath for the feet) described in a chapter **"5 Feet bath"** of the given book. However, for the people wishing by all means to get rid of the illness, following information is useful: A patient sick of depression and simultaneously of chronic fatigue syndrome cured by this method did feet bath (salt bath for the feet) the first month or one month and a half. Therefore, just in case, do feet bath (salt bath for the feet). Author of the given method (below, mostly "author") would recommend doing feet baths (salt baths for the feet) during the whole time of occupations by the method but not just month or one month and a half.

It makes sense to be occupied according to a chapter **"6 Part two of the universal method of drugless treatment for depression, chronic fatigue syndrome, other neurological diseases and hypertension"** of the present book instead of occupations according to the chapter **"3 Part one of the universal method of drugless treatment for depression, chronic fatigue syndrome, other neurological diseases and hypertension"** of the given book during 1-2 weeks (then, it is necessary to be occupied according to the chapter **"3 Part one of the universal method of drugless treatment for depression, chronic fatigue syndrome, other neurological diseases and hypertension"** of the present book 1-2 weeks again, then, to be occupied according to the chapter **"6 Part two of the universal method of drugless treatment for depression, chronic fatigue syndrome, other neurological diseases and hypertension"** of the given book 1-2 weeks again, etc.) only if occupations according to the chapter **"3 Part one of the universal method of drugless treatment for depression, chronic fatigue syndrome, other neurological diseases and hypertension"** of the present book become non-effective against your illness, i.e. if there is accustomization to occupations according to the chapter **"3 Part one of the universal method of drugless treatment for depression, chronic fatigue syndrome, other neurological diseases and hypertension"** of the given book.

2 General information

It should be mentioned that the present method was created exclusively with intention to help to people suffering from depression, however, it proved to be enough universal.

The example of a man sick of depression and simultaneously of chronic fatigue syndrome is characteristic. He was ill about four years and it was far not the first episode of this illness. Nobody was able to cure him. Depression is considered as one of the most poignant and hard to cure diseases. There is even an opinion that the one who will find a way of treatment for depression deserves the Nobel Prize (however, the present method cannot be nominated on the Nobel Prize, since it is not science-intensive, although, its simplicity and harmlessness are an advantage for the diseased ones). The author agrees with this opinion knowing about sufferings of the mentioned above person sick of depression. The statement of this person is characteristic: "Not everyone is capable to be kept from suicide at those sensations, which I experience". And really, many humans sick of depression commit suicide. It is known that depression and chronic fatigue syndrome are enough widespread diseases. For instance, 20-30 % of the population of our planet suffer from depression. In the case of this patient, there is a proof that just this method helped him. Feeling well enough, he has stopped to be engaged in it and he became bad in several days. He has resumed occupation by the method and he became again much better in two weeks. By the way, right at the beginning of occupation by the method he was engaged in it one and a half month for twenty minutes a day to overcome illness. Then, this patient began to be engaged for fifteen minutes daily. He began to be engaged for fifteen minutes right after he became good for the first time. After that, he tried to be engaged for five minutes but he became bad soon. At first, there was belief that such patients couldn't stop to be engaged in the method since etiology of this disease, most likely, is in genetics and it is necessary to be engaged daily and for enough time for counteraction to genetics omnipotent program. Anyway, if there is a desire to have a rest for several days or to interrupt occupation at all and if, as a result, there is the poor health it is necessary to recommence occupation. However, at the moment of last edition of the present book, aforementioned person sick of depression is not engaged in it already more than six years. However, his condition stabilized and, moreover, any traces of depression did not remain.

Occupation by the present method was accompanied by easy discomfort at the named patient but only at him and only during time of occupation (fifteen or twenty minutes a day), however, the end result says that the aim justifies the means. Therefore, there is a sense to follow the lead of this patient to people sick of depression and sick of chronic fatigue syndrome and also sick of these two illnesses simultaneously. It should be mentioned that this person sick of depression and simultaneously of chronic fatigue syndrome is quite weak-willed and the author had to tell him following every day: **"If occupations by this method for half a year will not help you will know, at least, that anything wouldn't help you".**

Among cured ones, there is also a woman who suffered from hypertension. The top pressure indication 180 and 200 was not rare for her. Even those preparations, which have been prescribed to her in several hospitals, which she laid for the last years in, did not help. The given method helped in two weeks of occupation according to its chapter **"3 Part one of the universal method of drugless treatment for depression, chronic fatigue syndrome, other neurological diseases and hypertension"** for ten minutes a day with position sitting on a chair or armchair. Now, pressure doesn't exceed norm. Unfortunately, the cessation of occupation led to return of high pressure in the case of the mentioned above woman.

Most probably, the suggested method is able to cure hypotension (low blood pressure) too. Hypotension is rare disease and, therefore, there are not concrete data concerning it yet.

Creation of the given method reminds known history of the invention of Galileo Galilei - a telescope. Galilei has guessed to bridge two lenses and a pipe in a single whole. The present method also successfully unites knowledge from different areas. And, despite it, it differs by very big and basic novelty. Full safety of the method is obvious as well.

It should be mentioned that some dilution of faeces, which start to remind infantile ones slightly that speaks about rejuvenating effect, is observed at all those engaged in the method. Therefore, most probably, the given method is capable to help to those ones suffering from constipation too. Supposition of the author that many other diseases can be cured too is based in considerable degree on that the offered method treats thanks just to the general rejuvenation of an organism.

According to the author's opinion, even each healthy person should be engaged in this method for very effective prophylaxis every year two weeks, which are apart for approximately or exactly half a year for ten-fifteen minutes a day.

If you are a diseased person, it is necessary to find from ten to fifty minutes a day (depending on your condition) for this method. If you consider necessary to find more than fifteen minutes a day for the method begin from fifteen minutes a day and add five minutes every week. If there is a possibility, engage in the method at the same time of days, it is better, according to alarm (clock) and not on a full stomach, i.e., basically, it is possible to be engaged just after awakening.

3 Part one of the universal method of drugless treatment for depression, chronic fatigue syndrome, other neurological diseases and hypertension

The given method represents absolutely special, including several very considerable know-hows auto-training in combination with dynamic exercises, which, as it is known, strengthen efficiency of auto-training. All know-hows are written by bold (heavy) type. The main know-hows are underlined thus too.

Author advises to pronounce all phrases of this auto-training in your native language. Even if you don't know the native language, author advises to find out how all phrases are pronounced in your native language, to remember all phrases and both each word and its meaning separately and to pronounce them when carrying out the method. The native language works much stronger.

The main phrases of this auto-training are following: "Yes, I shouldn't die", "Yes, I will live forever", "Yes, I take pleasure" and "Yes, I recover". It is necessary to tell these phrases by low whisper (perception by ears strengthens effect). Phrases are pronounced by turns. Each phrase or phrases united, as it is offered below, in pairs are pronounced with closed eyes approximately within forty five seconds (this term seems to be optimum, though, in each specific case, it can change according to your sensations, for example, according to disappearance of feeling of comfort at pronouncing the phrase or combination of phrases that is a signal to transition to other phrase). Basically, it is possible to unite phrases in pairs, for example, as follows: "Yes, I shouldn't die, yes, I will live forever" and "Yes, I take pleasure, yes, I recover". **However, it seems optimum pronouncing the first two phrases united together and pronouncing the last two phrases in separate way.** Sometimes, when the need is felt, the first two phrases can be pronounced not together but in separate way. **Anyway, it is desirable to pronounce, at least, the first two phrases advisably united together ("Yes, I shouldn't die, yes, I will live forever") with a sufficient share of panic and hysterics personifying your huge aspiration to recover (it is even much more pleasant than neutral intonation and in very many respects is the keystone to success). The people cured by the author pronounced these phrases just so.**

It seems to the author that following description of one person - his relative, the cousin grandmother - will help for realization of panic and hysterical intonation in optimum way. Author's cousin grandmother was dark-haired, rather thin than thick and of medium height. She had the higher medical education and worked as the laboratory assistant on research of results of medical analyses (of blood, etc.). She saw every day a huge number of microbes in a microscope and she treated in panic way to the fact if one didn't wash hands before taking food. She spoke in panic and hysterical thus: "Wash hands, wash hands". There was really so much panic and hysterics in it that I, at giving advices to my first patient – person sick of depression and simultaneously of chronic fatigue syndrome, cited an example of this woman whom he knew, and I pronounced two main phrases, it is desirable that united together ("Yes, I shouldn't die, yes, I will live forever"), of the method for this patient on native for the author and this patient Armenian language just with panic and hysterical and, besides, high (by thin voice) intonation of the cousin grandmother of the author. These two phrases united together

sound so in Armenian language: "Ha, es chi piti mernem, ha, es aprem havityan". In the word "piti" meaning "should", an accent should be done on the second syllable. In the word "aprem" meaning "will live", an accent should be done on the first syllable. In the word "havityan" meaning "forever", an accent should be done on the last syllable. However, the most important is that, copying the manner of the author's cousin grandmother, the author advised to his first patient sick of depression and simultaneously of chronic fatigue syndrome to do the general accent of these two phrases united together on the word "chi" meaning "not". Thus, this word is pronounced by more high-pitch tone (thinner voice) and in more panic and hysterical way than other words. It is necessary to explain meaning of two remaining words. "Ha" means "yes" and "es" means "I".

Photo of author's cousin grandmother in youth:

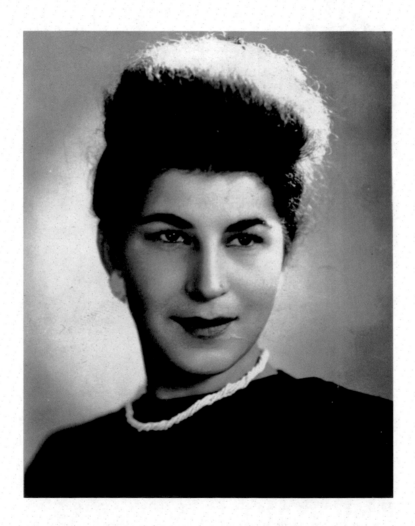

The author considers an image and intonation of his cousin grandmother as ideal ones for proper perception of how to pronounce two main united together phrases ("Yes, I shouldn't die, yes, I will live forever").

The key rule of any auto-training is concentration on sense of pronounced phrases. At the present auto-training, it is necessary to concentrate also on some parts of your body. For simplification of this problem, some movements will be offered far below too. **As to the first two phrases of the given auto-training ("Yes, I shouldn't die, yes, I will live forever"), at pronouncing them, it is necessary to realize (imagine) also at least by the edge of consciousness that, from all endocrine glands, the place of each of which, as it is known, coincides with corresponding to it chakra (chakras are spiritual and power centers along a backbone and in a head, they also are the pleasure centers (see the scheme of chakras not far below in the present chapter) except chakra Sahasrara (the place of Sahasrara doesn't have strict conformity to the endocrine gland, the place of the endocrine gland corresponding to this chakra coincides with the place of previous chakra - Agnya (Ajna) chakra), the hormones prolonging life are thrown out in a blood (it is necessary to imagine this).**

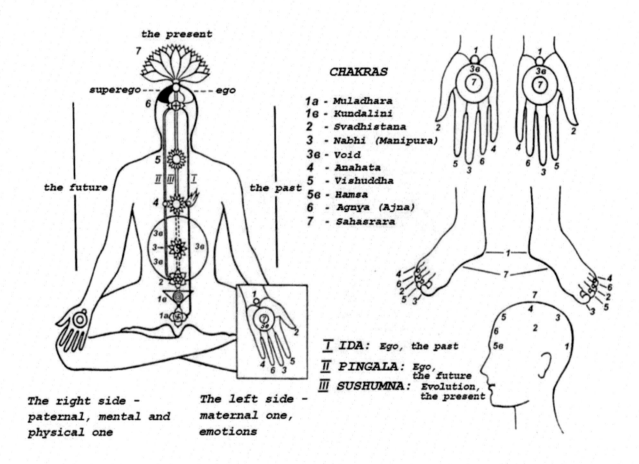

CHAKRAS

1a - Muladhara
1e - Kundalini
2 - Svadhistana
3 - Nabhi (Manipura)
3e - Void
4 - Anahata
5 - Vishuddha
5e - Hamsa
6 - Agnya (Ajna)
7 - Sahasrara

The right side - paternal, mental and physical one

The left side - maternal one, emotions

I IDA: Ego, the past
II PINGALA: Ego, the future
III SUSHUMNA: Evolution, the present

the present
superego --- ego
the future
the past

It is proved by scientists that the hormones secreted by endocrine glands regulate all functions of the organism including aging processes. In the book [13], [14], it is shown, that having achieved control over endocrine glands, it is possible to turn aging processes back. However, much less effective methods are offered in this book. It is known from the auto-training theory that both temporal shares of brain are involved at auto-training. Thus, it is a question of influence of one physical body (brain) on another (organism). It is a question in the book [13], [14], at best, of influence of thin bodies (aura) on the physical body (organism). It is clear that the latter doesn't stand up to comparison with the former.

The main know-how of the given method is expounded in the following paragraph:

Thus, positive action of the first two phrases of the offered method ("Yes, I shouldn't die, yes, I will live forever"), in case of many illnesses, can be explained by correctly picked

mechanism of influence on endocrine glands and, hence, on entire organism too. It is necessary to understand that the sense of these phrases represents only a key to this mechanism and it is necessary to pronounce them even if living for a long time doesn't enter into your plans. It is necessary to repeat that it is proved by scientists that the hormones secreted by glands regulate all functions of the organism including aging processes. The given mechanism of influence on endocrine glands and consequently on entire organism too uses a principle "by contradiction" (we influence on the organism by means of possibly even just artificially caused desire to live for a long time) that seems to be the only correct way. Continuing this thought, it is possible to confirm with the big share of probability that anything in the given method isn't casual and that, probably, it applies for soleness.

As it was mentioned above, it is known from the theory of auto-training that its action amplifies considerably at dynamic exercises. Therefore and for it would be easier to concentrate on the places of the organism corresponding to glands (on a vertical from the center of the head to the backbone bottom), it is necessary, sitting on the chair or on a floor in a pose Sukhasana (sit down on the floor, extend legs in front of yourself, bend the right leg having put the right foot under the left knee, bend the left leg and put the left foot under the right knee; the legs are crossed thus, however, they are not twisted in complicated way in a pretzel as in Lotus pose (Padmasana)), to make rockings of the top part of the body (from the bottom part of a back to the head inclusive; it is clear that the head makes movements with larger amplitude thus, while, the bottom part of the back is almost motionless) in a direction forward-back. At pronouncing the first phrase ("Yes, I shouldn't die"), it is necessary to do following additional movement too: It is necessary to shake the head negatively (as if saying "No" and despite the first word of the phrase is "Yes") and it is necessary to do it often and with small amplitude. However, it is necessary to notice that all present method including value of amplitudes of all movements should be edited by you depending on your desires. Regarding the first phrase, the author expects objection that the Universe doesn't hear a particle "…n't (not)" (the particle "…n't (not)" in this phrase is meant). Really, the particle "…n't (not)" itself is not audible to space, however, in the present method, the particle "Yes" is used before the particle "…n't (not)". The particle "Yes" as though sets the fashion on the general powerful and exclusively positive spirit and the particle "…n't (not)" in this case doesn't spoil a picture but quite the reverse. Positive results and absence of negative ones at people using this method testify to this. There are two more reasons speaking well for use of the particle "…n't (not)". The matter is that the second phrase ("Yes, I will live forever"), which in an optimum case is pronounced together with the first phrase ("Yes, I shouldn't die"), doesn't contain the particle "…n't (not)" and transformation of the first phrase, for example, in the following one: "Yes, I am immortal" in combination with the second phrase looks like something similar and, therefore, incorrect. One more reason speaking well for use of the particle "…n't (not)" is that this particle allows to add negative movements by the head (as if saying "No") too that promotes the best concentration on the brain and washing the brain and endocrine glands of the brain by blood. At pronouncing the second phrase ("…, yes, I will live forever"), it is necessary to do other additional movements. You should nod assent several times (as if saying "Yes"). **These nods assent (as if saying "Yes") as well as negative movements by the head (as if saying "No") too, besides psychological significance, help to concentrate better on the brain and head endocrine glands and to improve conditions of washing these glands by blood.** At pronouncing the first and second united phrases ("Yes, I shouldn't die, yes, I will live forever"), the head can be inclined slightly. At pronouncing the third and fourth phrases ("Yes, I take pleasure" and "Yes, I recover"), it is necessary, sitting on the chair or on the floor, to make rotary motions by a trunk and, as consequence, by the head with small amplitude. It is clear that, thus, the head makes movements with larger amplitude, while, the bottom part of the back is almost motionless. The head can be inclined slightly on one side thus. All it promotes concentration on the body and brain and promotes transformation of sense of the third and fourth phrases ("Yes, I take pleasure" and "Yes, I recover") in real sensations.

It is necessary to consider technique of pronouncing the phrases "Yes, I take pleasure" and "Yes, I recover" in more details. At pronouncing the first of the named phrases, it is necessary to try to imagine that information, in the form of pleasure (pleasant sensations), arrives from entire body or, at least, from entire brain on a hypothalamus (the pleasure center in the middle of the brain). It can turn out not at once. If it is impossible for a long time (a week) it is better not to point any more attention at pleasant sensations. It is enough that any sensations simply would be present and at any minimum volume. At pronouncing the phrase "Yes, I recover", it is necessary to try to feel that the information, in the form of the same pleasant sensations, spreads from the hypothalamus on entire brain or on entire body. It can turn out not at once too. If it is impossible for a long time (a week) it is better not to point any more attention at pleasant sensations. It is enough that any sensations simply would be present and at any minimum volume. However, it is necessary to mean that periodically repeating screwing up one's eyes promotes transformation of sense of the third phrase ("Yes, I take pleasure") in the real sensations corresponding to this sense (in pleasure). There is an opinion of scientists that essence of yoga is record of entire information about body on the hypothalamus (the pleasure center in the middle of the brain). There is also opinion of scientists that it leads to immortality. In the special literature, many people are listed, whose age exceeds one thousand and even two thousand years. It tells about presence of the big latent sense in pronouncing the third and fourth phrases, in doing the described far above in the present chapter movements accompanying them and, the main thing, in concentration on sensations arriving on the hypothalamus (the pleasure center in the middle of the brain) and on sensations spreading from it. Information of the present paragraph has almost the same importance as information of other paragraph adduced far above in the present chapter "3 Part one of the universal method of drugless treatment for depression, chronic fatigue syndrome, other neurological diseases and hypertension" and written in the same way, i.e. by bold (heavy) underlined type, since both these paragraphs concern the main know-hows of the present universal method.

In case of any serious diseases, it is possible to add the phrase referred on treatment for given concrete disease. For depression, chronic fatigue syndrome and simply for prophylaxis and self-improvement, it is possible to pronounce "Yes, my genetic program cardinally improves" and/or "Yes, I revive" (thus, it is desirable to imagine as the space between cells and genes is filled with vigorous energy). Such phrases can be not added but they can replace one of the third and fourth phrases or both the third and fourth phrases ("Yes, I take pleasure" and "Yes, I recover"). Most likely, it is necessary to do it not too often, since it is impossible to underestimate universality and, probably, indispensability of the first four phrases ("Yes, I shouldn't die", "Yes, I will live forever", "Yes, I take pleasure" and "Yes, I recover"). As to the mentioned above patient who has recovered from depression and chronic fatigue syndrome, he used only the phrase "Yes, my genetic program cardinally improves" sometimes.

It would be desirable to make recommendation, which, however, can be revised by you: Phrases "Yes, I shouldn't die" and "Yes, I will live forever" pronounced separately should occupy in sum not less than half of time of entire auto-training. If these phrases are united together, as it is recommended to make, their pronouncing should occupy not less than one third of time of entire auto-training.

There are days sometimes when pronouncing the above-mentioned phrases ("Yes, I shouldn't die, yes, I will live forever") seems to be as though too difficult. In such days, it is possible to pronounce any other phrases, which, it is desirable, should be directed on decision of any your problems too. There are days when you will want to pronounce phrases with open eyes. Basically, this desire can proceed several days successively or can be constant. Provided you are engaged long (30-50 minutes a day), necessity arises sometimes to interchange the positions of the phrases and movements for one day. Thus, the first two phrases ("Yes, I shouldn't die, yes, I will live forever") are pronounced at carrying out the movements corresponding to the third and fourth phrases ("Yes, I take pleasure" and "Yes, I recover"), and the third and fourth phrases ("Yes, I take pleasure" and "Yes, I recover") are pronounced at performance of the movements corresponding to the first and second phrases ("Yes, I shouldn't die, yes, I will live forever"). At pronouncing the first and second phrases ("Yes, I shouldn't die, yes, I will live forever"), affirmative and negative movements by the head can nevertheless be done if there is a desire.

Proceeding from previously named principle to be guided by your own desires, it is possible, at pronouncing any phrases, to do any elementary movements promoting concentration on the necessary places of the body. For example, the mentioned far above in the chapter **"2 General information"** of the present book and in the given chapter person to whom the present method has helped to recover from depression and chronic fatigue syndrome, at pronouncing all phrases always in the final stage of his occupations (the last month of the occupations), carried out only rotary motions by the trunk and, as consequence, by the head (it is clear that, thus, the head makes movements with larger amplitude, while, the bottom part of the back is almost motionless). The matter is that he felt giddy because of negative shakings by the head.

As it was mentioned above, it is necessary to find from ten to fifty minutes a day for the present method and, it is desirable, at the same time of days. Entire occupation or its first minutes can be spent sitting on the chair or armchair or sitting on the floor in the elementary pose of yoga – the pose Sukhasana (sit down on the floor, extend legs in front of yourself, bend the right leg having put the right foot under the left knee, bend the left leg and put the left foot under the right knee; the legs are crossed thus, however, they are not twisted in complicated way in a pretzel as in Lotus pose (Padmasana)). Sometimes, the pose Sukhasana (sit down on the floor, extend legs in front of yourself, bend the right leg having put the right foot under the left knee, bend the left leg and put the left foot under the right knee; the legs are crossed thus, however, they are not twisted in complicated way in a pretzel as in Lotus pose (Padmasana)) can be changed for a short while to the pose Vajarasana (it is similar to the pose of the praying Moslem, however, one should hold the back upright always). It is necessary to repeat and generalize the idea stated earlier that choice of the moment of transition from one pose and/or type of movements and/or phrase to other pose and/or type of movements and/or phrase should be done guiding by condition of disappearance of feeling of comfort at carrying out any certain pose and/or type of movements and/or phrase that is a signal to its/their change.

Instructions mostly concerning occupation in lying position follow below in the present chapter, however, as to the mentioned above person who has recovered from depression, he never was engaged in lying position but he alternated the pose Sukhasana (sit down on the floor, extend legs in front of yourself, bend the right leg having put the right foot under the left knee, bend the left leg and put the left foot under the right knee; the legs are crossed thus, however, they are not twisted in complicated way in a pretzel as in Lotus pose (Padmasana)) with sitting on the chair and the mentioned above woman, which has recovered from hypertension, was engaged on the chair or in the armchair always. It should be mentioned that the main pose for meditation is the sitting position. The author believes that it is not casually. Therefore, who has possibility to be engaged being sitting let him/her be engaged being sitting, while, the lying positions are intended mostly for those who cannot be engaged being sitting and for those who is engaged more than fifteen-twenty minutes, which, by the way, are desirable for spending, as far as possible, in one or several sitting positions. Thus, it is possible to use the last minutes of occupation, which follow first fifteen-twenty minutes spent in one or several sitting positions, as follows: It is necessary to lie down on the floor covered with a carpet or laying (thin carpet) on one's right side and to close eyes. The left hand should be raised upwards and one has to make rotary motions with small amplitude by it. It is possible to put the right hand under the head or to put it on the floor or to raise slightly without tearing off the right shoulder from the floor. As option: It is possible to extend both hands over the head either parallel to longitudinal axis of the body or nearly so being as though extending and increasing height (if you would stand thus you would reach for a ceiling). The right hand can be motionless, while, the left one can make movements extending height (it is possible to do it beginning from initial vertical position of this hand), or it can make rotary motions with small amplitude as it has been told above. Also, the hands can be bent in elbows being connected by palms. The head can be put on the right forearm sometimes. It is necessary to turn over on one's left side after approximately two minutes. Thus, it is necessary to raise upwards the right hand making by it rotary motions with small amplitude. It is possible to put the right hand under the head or to put it on the floor either to raise it slightly without tearing off the left shoulder from the floor. As option: It is possible to extend both hands over the head either parallel to longitudinal axis of the body or nearly so being as though extending and increasing height (if you would stand thus you would reach for the ceiling). The left hand can be motionless, while, the right one can make either movements increasing height or it can make rotary motions with small amplitude as it has been told above. Also, the hands can be bent in elbows being connected by palms. The head can be put on the left forearm sometimes. Approximately in two minutes, it is necessary to lie down on the back, to raise upwards both hands making by them rotary motions with small amplitude, it is possible, to the opposite directions. Basically, it is possible to make, by the hands, from their initial vertical position, movements increasing height. Lying on the back, it is possible to bend legs in knees (in this case, feet occur on the floor) sometimes and to remain in this pose continuing to do all as it is described above. As option: It is possible to lie down on a breast and to extend both hands over the head either parallel to longitudinal axis of the body or nearly so being as though extending and increasing height (if you would stand thus you would reach for the ceiling). Also, the hands can be bent in elbows being connected by palms. At occupation being lying, it is necessary to pronounce the phrases of the suggested auto-training by low whisper too. If it is inconveniently to do thus such movements as negative and affirmative ones by the head it is possible not to do them. At occupation being lying, it is inexpedient to achieve constant conformity of poses to phrases.

Proceeding from previously named principle to be guided by desires, it is possible, to alternate, several times, occupation sitting on the chair and/or in the pose Sukhasana (sit down on the floor, extend legs in front of yourself, bend the right leg having put the right foot under the left knee, bend the left leg and put the left foot under the right knee; the legs are crossed thus, however, they are not twisted in complicated way in a pretzel as in Lotus pose (Padmasana)) and/or in the pose Vajarasana (it is similar to the pose of the praying Moslem, however, one should hold the back upright always) to occupation in lying position. Time spent in occupation sitting on the chair and/or in the pose Sukhasana (sit down on the floor, extend legs in front of yourself, bend the right leg having put the right foot under the left knee, bend the left leg and put the left foot under the right knee; the legs are crossed thus, however, they are not twisted in complicated way in a pretzel as in Lotus pose (Padmasana)) and/or in the pose Vajarasana (it is similar to the pose of the praying Moslem, however, one should hold the back upright always) and in occupation in lying position can be different. For example, occupation can be constructed as follows: It is necessary to use the following types of movements having been already considered far above and above in the present chapter (we will begin with movements in any of sitting positions and let's name them "the first type of movements"): As it was mentioned far above in the present chapter **"3 Part one of the universal method of drugless treatment for depression, chronic fatigue syndrome, other neurological diseases and hypertension"**, each phrase of auto-training or two its phrases, which were recommended to be united ("Yes, I shouldn't die, yes, I will live forever"), should correspond to each type of movements in the sitting position on the chair and/or in the pose Sukhasana (sit down on the floor, extend legs in front of yourself, bend the right leg having put the right foot under the left knee, bend the left leg and put the left foot under the right knee; the legs are crossed thus, however, they are not twisted in complicated way in a pretzel as in Lotus pose (Padmasana)) and/ or in the pose Vajarasana (it is similar to the pose of the praying Moslem, however, one should hold the back upright always). It is necessary to remind the first type of movements, which two named united phrases correspond to: It is necessary to sit on the chair or in the pose Sukhasana (sit down on the floor, extend legs in front of yourself, bend the right leg having put the right foot under the left knee, bend the left leg and put the left foot under the right knee; the legs are crossed thus, however, they are not twisted in complicated way in a pretzel as in Lotus pose (Padmasana)) either in the pose Vajarasana (it is similar to the pose of the praying Moslem, however, one should hold the back upright always) and it is necessary to make rockings by the trunk and, as consequence, by the head in a direction forward-back. It is clear that, thus, the head makes movements with larger amplitude, while, the bottom part of the back is almost motionless. At pronouncing the first of two above-mentioned united phrases ("Yes, I shouldn't die"), it is necessary to do following additional movement too: It is necessary to shake the head negatively (as if saying "No" and despite the first word of the phrase is "Yes") and to do it often and with small amplitude (however, it is necessary to notice once again that all present method including value of amplitudes of all movements should be edited by you depending on your desires). At pronouncing the second phrase ("Yes, I will live forever"), it is necessary to do other additional movement: You should nod assent several times (as if saying "Yes"). These additional movements, besides psychological significance, help to concentrate better on the head endocrine glands and to improve conditions of washing these endocrine glands by blood. At pronouncing the first and second phrases ("Yes, I shouldn't die, yes, I will live forever"), the head can be inclined slightly. The second type of movements, which the third phrase "Yes, I take pleasure" corresponds to, is following: It is necessary to lie down on the floor covered with the carpet or laying (thin carpet) on one's right side and to close eyes. The left hand should be raised upwards and one has to make rotary motions with small amplitude by it. It is possible to put the right hand under the head or to put it on the floor either to raise it slightly without tearing off the right shoulder from the floor. As option: It is possible to extend both hands over the head either parallel to longitudinal axis of the body or nearly so being as though extending and increasing height (if you would stand thus you would reach for the ceiling). The right hand can be motionless, while, the left one can make movements extending height (it is possible to do it beginning from initial vertical position of this hand) or it can make rotary motions with small amplitude as it has been told above. Also, the hands can be bent in elbows being connected by palms. The head can be put on the right forearm sometimes. The third type of movements, which the fourth phrase corresponds to "Yes, I recover", is following: It is necessary to lie down on the floor covered with the carpet or laying (thin carpet) on one's left side and to close eyes. The right hand should be raised upwards and one has to make rotary motions with small amplitude by it. It is possible to put the left hand under the head or to put it on the floor either to raise it slightly without tearing off the left shoulder from the floor. As option: It is possible to extend both hands over the head either parallel to longitudinal axis of the body or nearly so being as though extending and increasing height (if you would stand thus you would reach for the ceiling). The left hand can be motionless, while, the right one can make either movements increasing height or it can make rotary motions with small amplitude as it has been told above. Also, the hands can be bent in elbows being connected by palms. The head can be put on the left forearm sometimes.

Basically, it is possible to add three more following types of movements, which as well as the ones considered above have been already mentioned in the present chapter **"3 Part one of the universal method of drugless treatment for depression, chronic fatigue syndrome, other neurological diseases and hypertension"**:

The fourth type of movements: It is necessary to lie down on the back, to raise upwards both hands making by them rotary motions with small amplitude, it is possible, to the opposite directions. Basically, it is possible to make movements by the hands increasing height (if you would stand thus you would reach for the ceiling). Lying on the back, it is possible to bend, sometimes, legs in knees (the feet are on the floor thus) and to remain in this pose continuing to do all as it is described above. As option: It is possible to lie down on the breast and to extend both hands over the head either parallel to longitudinal axis of the body or nearly so being as though extending and increasing height (if you would stand thus you would reach for the ceiling). Also, the hands can be bent in elbows being connected by palms. The fifth type of movements: It is necessary sitting on the chair or on the floor in the pose Sukhasana (sit down on the floor, extend legs in front of yourself, bend the right leg having put the right foot under the left knee, bend the left leg and put the left foot under the right knee; the legs are crossed thus, however, they are not twisted in complicated way in a pretzel as in Lotus pose (Padmasana)), to make rotary motions by a trunk and, as consequence, by the head with small amplitude. It is clear that the head makes movements with larger amplitude thus, while, the bottom part of the back is almost motionless. The head can be inclined slightly on one side thus. The sixth type of movements: Make the same movements, however, sitting in the pose Vajarasana (it is similar to the pose of the praying Moslem, however, one should hold the back upright always). As you understand, then, it is necessary to pass again to the first type of movements, then, to the second one and so on. If any type of movements represents difficulty it is necessary to exclude it.

It is clear that, at addition of the first three types of movements or, at least, of one of them, pronouncing the united phrases "Yes, I shouldn't die, yes, I will live forever" will not always correspond to the first type of movements. The first type of movements is intended, as a matter of fact, just for these phrases. Therefore, the first type of movements, in this case, should be used only in need of pronouncing these phrases in sitting position. At pronouncing other phrases in sitting position, it is necessary to replace the first type of movements by the fifth or sixth types of movements.

It should be mentioned that, as a matter of fact, the offered method comes to carrying out several simple movements, to pronouncing several phrases and to concentration on sense of phrases, on a vertical from the brain to a tailbone, in which area endocrine glands (endocrine glands are located also in the brain) are located, to concentration on the brain and on the trunk. Some significance belongs to correct synchronism of carrying out movements and pronouncing phrases.

The author told to all the patients that it is possible to learn phrases, movements and internal imaginations of this method within several minutes and the method began to seem to them simple and effective instantly.

Important advice: It is not recommended to drink even light alcoholic drinks. Some undesirable reaction, besides, rejecting back on several parameters, takes place.

4 Keys to the method

Author considers as the main key to the method following information: **The method is constructed on logic of treatment of depression only but it proved to be enough universal. Author advises to track logic of treatment for depression in the chapter "3 Part one of the universal method of drugless treatment for depression, chronic fatigue syndrome, other neurological diseases and hypertension" of the present book.** The appropriate paragraphs from the chapter "**3 Part one of the universal method of drugless treatment for depression, chronic fatigue syndrome, other neurological diseases and hypertension**" of the present book required to track logic of treatment are adduced as follows for your convenience:

It is proved by scientists that the hormones secreted by endocrine glands regulate all functions of the organism including aging processes. In the book [13], [14], it is shown, that having achieved control over endocrine glands, it is possible to turn aging processes back. However, much less effective methods are offered in this book. It is known from the auto-training theory that both temporal shares of brain are involved at auto-training. Thus, it is a question of influence of one physical body (brain) on another (organism). It is a question in the book [13], [14], at best, of influence of thin bodies (aura) on the physical body (organism). It is clear that the latter doesn't stand up to comparison with the former.

The main know-how of the present universal method is adduced in the following paragraph:

<u>Thus, positive action of the first two phrases of the offered method ("Yes, I shouldn't die, yes, I will live forever"), in case of many illnesses, can be explained by correctly picked mechanism of influence on endocrine glands and, hence, on entire organism too. It is necessary to understand that the sense of these phrases represents only a key to this mechanism and it is necessary to pronounce them even if living for a long time doesn't enter into your plans. It is necessary to repeat that it is proved by scientists that the hormones secreted by glands regulate all functions of the organism including aging processes. The given mechanism of influence on endocrine glands and consequently on entire organism too uses a principle "by contradiction" (we influence on the organism by means of possibly even just artificially caused desire to live for a long time) that seems to be the only correct way. Continuing this thought, it is possible to confirm with the big share of probability that anything in the given method isn't casual and that, probably, it applies for soleness.</u>

Other important information from the chapter "**3 Part one of the universal method of drugless treatment for depression, chronic fatigue syndrome, other neurological diseases and hypertension**" of the present book is adduced as follows for your convenience:

The key rule of any auto-training is concentration on sense of pronounced phrases. At the given auto-training, it is necessary to concentrate also on some parts of your body. For simplification of this problem, some movements will be offered far below too. **As to the first two phrases of the given auto-training ("Yes, I shouldn't die, yes, I will live forever"), at pronouncing them, it is necessary to realize (imagine) also at least by the edge of consciousness that from all endocrine glands, the place of each of which, as it is known, coincides with corresponding to it chakra (chakras are spiritual and power centers along a backbone and in a head, they also are the pleasure centers (see the scheme of chakras not far below and on the last page of the given document) except chakra Sahasrara (the place of Sahasrara doesn't have strict conformity to the** endocrine gland, the place of the endocrine gland corresponding to this chakra coincides with the place of previous chakra - Agnya (Ajna) chakra), the hormones prolonging life are thrown out in a blood (it is necessary to imagine this).

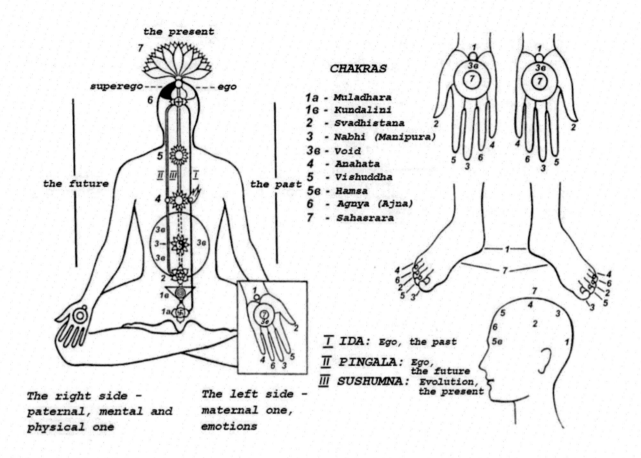

CHAKRAS

1a - Muladhara
1в - Kundalini
2 - Svadhistana
3 - Nabhi (Manipura)
3в - Void
4 - Anahata
5 - Vishuddha
5в - Hamsa
6 - Agnya (Ajna)
7 - Sahasrara

the present

the future   the past

superego ---- ego

The right side - paternal, mental and physical one

The left side - maternal one, emotions

I   IDA: Ego, the past
II PINGALA: Ego, the future
III SUSHUMNA: Evolution, the present

The second main know-how of the present universal method is adduced in the following paragraph:

It is necessary to consider technique of pronouncing the phrases "Yes, I take pleasure" and "Yes, I recover" in more details. At pronouncing the first of the named phrases, it is necessary to try to imagine that information, in the form of pleasure (pleasant sensations), arrives from entire body or, at least, from entire brain on a hypothalamus (the pleasure center in the middle of the brain). It can turn out not at once. If it is impossible for a long time (a week) it is better not to point any more attention at pleasant sensations. It is enough that any sensations simply would be present and at any minimum volume. At pronouncing the phrase "Yes, I recover", it is necessary to try to feel that the information, in the form of the same pleasant sensations, spreads from the hypothalamus on entire brain or on entire body. It can turn out not at once too. If it is impossible for a long time (a week) it is better not to point any more attention at pleasant sensations. It is enough that any sensations simply would be present and at any minimum volume. However, it is necessary to mean that periodically repeating screwing up one's eyes promotes transformation of sense of the third phrase ("Yes, I take pleasure") in the real sensations corresponding to this sense (in pleasure).

There is an opinion of scientists that essence of yoga is record of entire information about body on the hypothalamus (the pleasure center in the middle of the brain). There is also opinion of scientists that it leads to immortality. In the special literature, many people are listed, whose age exceeds one thousand and even two thousand years. It tells about presence of the big latent sense in pronouncing the third and fourth phrases, in doing the described far above in the present chapter movements accompanying them and, the main thing, in concentration on sensations arriving on the hypothalamus (the pleasure center in the middle of the brain) and on sensations spreading from it. Information of the present paragraph has almost the same importance as information of other paragraph adduced far above in the present chapter "4 Keys to the method" and in the chapter "3 Part one of the universal method of drugless treatment for depression, chronic fatigue syndrome, other neurological diseases and hypertension" of the present book and written in the same way, i.e. by bold (heavy) underlined type, since both these paragraphs concern the main know-hows of the present universal method.

5 Feet bath

Basically, you can not do feet bath (salt bath for the feet) at all. However, for the people wishing to get rid of the illness by all means, following information is useful: The patient sick of depression and simultaneously of chronic fatigue syndrome cured by this method did feet bath (salt bath for the feet) during the first month or one month and a half of occupations. Therefore, if you are sick of depression and simultaneously of chronic fatigue syndrome, just in case, do feet bath (salt bath for the feet). The author recommends doing feet baths (salt baths for the feet) during the whole time of occupations by the method but not just month or one month and a half. Therefore, it makes sense to adduce recommendations concerning the feet bath (salt bath for the feet) from Russian version of published not by publishing house but by enthusiasts of Sahaja yoga "Methodic textbook for beginners" (on Sahaja yoga; Sahaja yoga is recognized all over the world metascience directed at optimization of opening chakras process, however, it represents, in fact, non-pleasant actions, which should last approximately two years of twice a day repetitions each of at least half an hour's duration for to open at least one chakra) (this "Methodic textbook…" is written in Russian and, therefore, just several its needed fragments are translated and adduced in the present book), it makes sense to describe how the patient sick of depression and simultaneously of chronic fatigue syndrome did the feet bath (salt bath for the feet) and, also, it makes sense to describe how the author did the feet bath (salt bath for the feet). Thus, recommendations concerning the feet bath (salt bath for the feet) from Russian version of published not by publishing house but by enthusiasts of Sahaja yoga "Methodic textbook for beginners" (on Sahaja yoga) are as follows: "Before evening meditation, it is good to apply the feet bath *(salt bath for the feet)* (use water of comfortable temperature, a water level - on an ankle, salt – 1-2 table spoons) within 10 minutes. Then, it is necessary to rinse feet by pure water, to pour out water from a basin in a toilet and to wash up hands. It is very effective technique of removal of negativity through water and earth elements (salt is an earth element)". Difference of a way of use of the feet bath (salt bath for the feet) by the patient sick of depression and simultaneously of chronic fatigue syndrome is as follows: This person made the feet bath (salt bath for the feet) not before occupation by the given method but simultaneously with this occupation and as long as it lasted. As it has been told in the chapter **"3 Part one of the universal method of drugless treatment for depression, chronic fatigue syndrome, other neurological diseases and hypertension"** of the present book, this patient seriously sick of depression and simultaneously of chronic fatigue syndrome was engaged for 20 minutes a day in the beginning and, then, - for 15 minutes. In a month – one and a half month, he stopped to do the feet baths (salt baths for the feet) but continued to be engaged in the given method. The author possesses his own experience in doing feet baths (salt baths for the feet) in context of occupations only according to the chapter **"4 The second method of drugless deliverance from dropping-off to sleep disorder"** of Part 1 **"The four most effective methods of deliverance from insomnia, three of which permit to manage without soporific"** of the present book. Nevertheless, following recommendations of the author concerning the feet baths (salt baths for the feet) are relevant: It is possible to use both the rock-salt and any sea one. If you use the deep basin (such basins are plastic ones in majority of cases) it is necessary to put into the basin not two spoons of salt as it is told in published not by publishing house but by enthusiasts of Sahaja yoga "Methodic textbook for beginners" (on Sahaja yoga) but four spoons of salt. The author used to put, in the deep basin, three spoons of sea salt with the top (i.e. as much as the spoon is able to contain), one spoon of the rock-salt with the top and mixed water before full dissolution of salt. As regards sea salt, it is usually on sale in drugstores. Salt of ancient sea is preferable. The author liked to provide water temperature in the basin, in the beginning of occupation (before pouring salt), 35-36 degrees Celsius, it is desirable, not more and not less. At the subsequent period of occupation, the author had a desire to reduce water temperature in the basin, in the beginning of occupation (before pouring salt), to 34 degrees Celsius exactly. You should not exceed time of occupation with use of the feet bath (salt bath for the feet) in 30-35 minutes.

It is possible to do the feet bath (salt bath for the feet) both during occupation according to the chapter **"3 Part one of the universal method of drugless treatment for depression, chronic fatigue syndrome, other neurological diseases and hypertension"** or the chapter **"6 Part two of the universal method of drugless treatment for depression, chronic fatigue syndrome, other neurological diseases and hypertension"** of the present book and after occupation according to the chapter **"3 Part one of the universal method of drugless treatment for depression, chronic fatigue syndrome, other neurological diseases and hypertension"** or the chapter **"6 Part two of the universal method of drugless treatment for depression, chronic fatigue syndrome, other neurological diseases and hypertension"** of the present book, however, you should not exceed time of occupation with use of the feet bath (salt bath for the feet) in 30-35 minutes in any case.

6 Part two of the universal method of drugless treatment for depression, chronic fatigue syndrome, other neurological diseases and hypertension

In the course of occupation according to the chapter **"3 Part one of the universal method of drugless treatment for depression, chronic fatigue syndrome, other neurological diseases and hypertension"** of the present book, person who suffered from depression and chronic fatigue syndrome and who was cured by the present method felt bad again (it happened before his condition stabilized, i.e. before he ceased to be engaged in the method). Then, the author advised to him to be engaged in other kind of auto-training. And it worked approximately a week later. The patient felt better. **The conclusion arises: If accustomization to occupations according to the chapter "3 Part one of the universal method of drugless treatment for depression, chronic fatigue syndrome, other neurological diseases and hypertension" of the present book is observed, it is necessary to start being engaged according to the given chapter "6 Part two of the universal method of drugless treatment for depression, chronic fatigue syndrome, other neurological diseases and hypertension" of the present book and to do it 1-2 weeks, then, it is necessary to be engaged 1-2 weeks according to the chapter "3 Part one of the universal method of drugless treatment for depression, chronic fatigue syndrome, other neurological diseases and hypertension" of the given book again, then again, it is necessary to be engaged according to the present chapter "6 Part two of the universal method of drugless treatment for depression, chronic fatigue syndrome, other neurological diseases and hypertension" of the present book 1-2 weeks, etc.**

The mentioned closer to the beginning of the present chapter **"6 Part two of the universal method of drugless treatment for depression, chronic fatigue syndrome, other neurological diseases and hypertension"** another kind of auto-training is adopted by the author with some changes from Sahaja yoga. It is necessary to pay attention only on the end of the third page, on the entire fourth page of the published not by publishing house but by enthusiasts of Sahaja yoga "Methodic textbook for beginners" (on Sahaja yoga) (see heading **"Assertions for rise of Kundalini"** of the translated information from the mentioned methodic textbook adduced far below in the present chapter **"6 Part two of the universal method of drugless treatment for depression, chronic fatigue syndrome, other neurological diseases and hypertension"** and text below this heading) and on the beginning of the seventh page (see heading **"Assertions for the central channel"** of the translated information from the published not by publishing house but by enthusiasts of Sahaja yoga "Methodic textbook for beginners" (on Sahaja yoga) adduced far below in the present chapter **"6 Part two of the universal method of drugless treatment for depression, chronic fatigue syndrome, other neurological diseases and hypertension"** and text below this heading).

Thus, all necessary information from published not by publishing house but by enthusiasts of Sahaja yoga "Methodic textbook for beginners" (on Sahaja yoga) is adduced as follows:

Reference information from the very beginning of published not by publishing house but by enthusiasts of Sahaja yoga "Methodic textbook for beginners" (on Sahaja yoga) is as follows:

"You can't learn value of your life until you aren't connected to that force which has created you".

Shri Mataji Nirmala Devi

Sahaja yoga

On May 5, 1970, Shri Mataji Nirmala Devi opened to the world a sacral way of the spiritual ascension named "Sahaja yoga". The word "Sahaja" means "innate" and "yoga" is "union" of our inner self with All-penetrating Energy - energy of love and the compassion piercing each atom of the Universe. For realization of this union, there is energy named "Kundalini" (translation of this word from Sanskrit is "rolled up by a spiral", it is rolled into 3.5 turns) in our sacral bone "sacrum". This potential energy put in us since the birth is similar to the potential energy of the big tree put in a small seed. Awakening Kundalini is a shoot of this seed, beginning of the way to full Self-realization – to realizing by the person of his true "I".

Information from the end of the third page and from entire fourth page of published not by publishing house but by enthusiasts of Sahaja yoga "Methodic textbook for beginners" (on Sahaja yoga) is as follows:

Assertions for rise of Kundalini

Sit down conveniently. The left hand symbolizing desire put on a knee with a palm "looking" upwards, in a direction to a portrait of Shri Mataji. Move the right hand on left-hand side of a body according to drawings.

Address can be such: "Mother, …" or "Shri Mataji, …". When you pronounce assertions, do all sincerely, with all your heart, not mechanically.

1

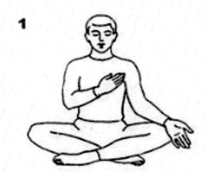

The right hand is on a heart. Ask a question in your heart three times: *"Mother, am I a Spirit?"*

2

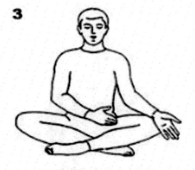

The right hand is in the top part of a stomach, under ribs. Ask 3 times: *"Mother, am I a teacher for myself?"*

3

The right hand is on the bottom part of the stomach (the left groin). Ask sincerely 6 times: *"Mother, please, give me pure Knowledge".*

4

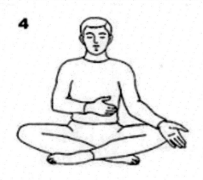

The right hand comes back to the top part of the stomach. Tell in the affirmative 10 times: *"Mother, I am the teacher for myself".*

5

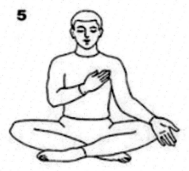

The right hand is on the heart. Here, tell 12 times affirmatively, with full confidence: *"Mother, I am the Spirit".*

6

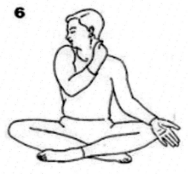

Put the right hand on a corner between a neck and the left shoulder, turn the head to the right and tell 16 times in the affirmative, without sense of guilt: *"Mother, I am not guilty in anything".*

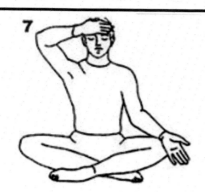

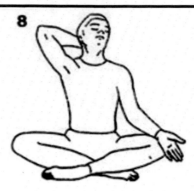

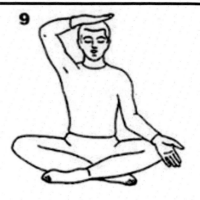

7 Put the right hand on a forehead, press densely and incline the head forward. Tell (it is not important how many times): *"Mother, I forgive everybody"*. Forgive everybody sincerely, with all your heart.

8 Put the right hand on a back of the head, throw back your head. Tell: *"Mother, please, forgive me if I have made any mistakes voluntarily or not"*.

9 Put the right hand by the palm center on a top of the head, move fingers apart and make effort to direct (bend) them upwards. Having pressed a palm strongly, rotate it together with a head skin 7 times clockwise each time applying: *"Mother, please, give me Self-realization"*.

Information from the beginning of the seventh page of published not by publishing house but by enthusiasts of Sahaja yoga "Methodic textbook for beginners" (on Sahaja yoga) is as follows:

Assertions for the central channel

Pronouncing assertions address in following way: "Mother, …" or "Shri Matadzhi, …"

1. Muladhara – please, make me innocent.

2. Svadhistana – please, make me the creative person.

3. Nabhi (Manipura) – please, give me spiritual satisfaction.
   3a. Void - please, make me the teacher for myself.

4. Anahata – please, make me the fearless person.

5. Vishuddha - please, make me the collective person.
   5a. Hamsa - please, make me the acute person, capable to distinguish the good from the bad.

6. Agnya (Ajna) - please, make me the forgiving person.

7. Sahasrara – please, strengthen my Self-realization.

Mentioned many times far above in the present Part 2 **"Universal method of drugless treatment for depression, chronic fatigue syndrome, other neurological diseases and hypertension"** of the given book person who suffered from depression and chronic fatigue syndrome practised mostly the assertions adduced in the end of the third page and on entire fourth page of published not by publishing house but by enthusiasts of Sahaja yoga "Methodic textbook for beginners" (on Sahaja yoga) (see far above in the present chapter **"6 Part two of the universal method of drugless treatment for depression, chronic fatigue syndrome, other neurological diseases and hypertension"** nine illustrations of a human carrying out Sahaja yoga and see inscriptions under each illustration) in full conformity with the instructions given to each assertion (inscriptions under each illustration). The change brought by the author consists in that, according to Sahaja yoga, the given assertions were supposed to be said only once at the very beginning of occupation by this discipline, while, the author has suggested to pronounce these assertions within all fifteen minutes of daily occupation. However, approximately, one time in four days, the person who suffered from depression and chronic fatigue syndrome practised the assertions adduced in the beginning of the seventh page of published not by publishing house but by enthusiasts of Sahaja yoga "Methodic textbook for beginners" (on Sahaja yoga) (see text far above in the present chapter **"6 Part two of the universal method of drugless treatment for depression, chronic fatigue syndrome, other neurological diseases and hypertension"** after heading **"Assertions for the central channel"**). He pronounced each assertion approximately for forty five seconds that seemed him optimum. In both cases, he pronounced assertions in a whisper but he didn't do any movements, which are recommended in the chapter **"3 Part one of the universal method of drugless treatment for depression, chronic fatigue syndrome, other neurological diseases and hypertension"** of the present book.

Any of patients of the author didn't do dynamic exercises at occupations according to the given chapter **"6 Part two of the universal method of drugless treatment for depression, chronic fatigue syndrome, other neurological diseases and hypertension"**, however, taking into consideration ability of dynamic exercises to strengthen efficiency of auto-training, there is a sense at least to try to do any movements. It seems optimum to do five following types of movements (all of them on the whole coincide with movements suggested in chapter **"3 Part one of the universal method of drugless treatment for depression, chronic fatigue syndrome, other neurological diseases and hypertension"** of the present book), each of these movements should correspond to each regular assertion: The first type of movements: It is necessary, sitting on the chair or on the floor in the pose Sukhasana (sit down on the floor, extend legs in front of yourself, bend the right leg having put the right foot under the left knee, bend the left leg and put the left foot under the right knee; the legs are crossed thus, however, they are not twisted in complicated way in a pretzel as in Lotus pose (Padmasana)), to make rotary motions by the trunk and, as consequence, by the head with small amplitude. It is clear that the head makes movements with larger amplitude thus, while, the bottom part of the back is almost motionless. The head can be inclined slightly on one side thus. The second type of movements: Make the same movements, however, sitting in the pose Vajarasana (it is similar to the pose of the praying Moslem, however, one should hold the back upright always). The third type of movements: It is necessary to lie down on the floor covered with the carpet or laying (thin carpet) on one's right side and to close eyes. The left hand should be raised upwards and one has to make rotary motions with small amplitude by it. It is possible to put the right hand under the head or to put it on the floor either to raise it slightly without tearing off the right shoulder from the floor. As option: It is possible to extend both hands over the head either parallel to longitudinal axis of the body or nearly so being as though extending and increasing height (if you would stand thus you would reach for a ceiling). The right hand can be motionless, while, the left one can make movements extending height (it is possible to do it beginning from initial vertical position of this hand) or it can make rotary motions with small amplitude as it has been told above. Also, the hands can be bent in elbows being connected by palms. The head can be put on the right forearm sometimes. The fourth type of movements: It is necessary to lie down on the floor covered with the carpet or laying (thin carpet) on one's left side and to close eyes. The right hand should be raised upwards and one has to make rotary motions with small amplitude by it. It is possible to put the left hand under the head or to put it on the floor either to raise it slightly without tearing off the left shoulder from the floor. It is possible to extend both hands over the head either parallel to longitudinal axis of the body or nearly so being as though extending and increasing height (if you would stand thus you would reach for a ceiling). The left hand can be motionless, while, the right one can make either movements extending growth (it is possible to do it beginning from initial vertical position of this hand) or it can make rotary motions with small amplitude as it has been told above. Also, the hands can be bent in elbows being connected by palms. The head can be put on the left forearm sometimes. The fifth type of movements: It is necessary to lie down on the back, to raise upwards both hands making by them rotary motions with small amplitude, it is possible, to the opposite directions. Basically, it is possible to make, by the hands, from their initial vertical position, movements extending height. Lying on the back, it is possible to bend, sometimes, legs in knees (the feet are on the floor thus) and to remain in this pose continuing to do all as it is described above. As option: It is possible to lie down on the breast and to extend both hands over the head either parallel to longitudinal axis of the body or nearly so being as though extending and increasing height (if you would stand thus you would reach for the ceiling). Also, the hands can be bent in elbows being connected by palms. As you understand, then, it is necessary to pass again to the first type of movements, then, to the second one and so on. If any type of movements represents difficulty it is necessary to exclude it.

There is some theoretical probability that there will be accustomization to occupations according to the chapters **"3 Part one of the universal method of drugless treatment for depression, chronic fatigue syndrome, other neurological diseases and hypertension"** and **"6 Part two of the universal method of drugless treatment for depression, chronic fatigue syndrome, other neurological diseases and hypertension"** of the present book. Therefore, if there is such necessity, the assertions adduced in the beginning of the seventh page of published not by publishing house but by enthusiasts of Sahaja yoga "Methodic textbook for beginners" (on Sahaja yoga) (see heading **"Assertions for rise of Kundalini"** of the translated information from the mentioned methodic textbook adduced far above in the present chapter **"6 Part two of the universal method of drugless treatment for depression, chronic fatigue syndrome, other neurological diseases and hypertension"** and text below this heading) could be considered as independent auto-training, the third in succession, i.e. it is not necessary to be engaged in it before there is such need. Basically, it is possible to invent other assertions too. A key rule: **If accustomization to occupations according to the chapter "3 Part one of the universal method of drugless treatment for depression, chronic fatigue syndrome, other neurological diseases and hypertension" of the present book is observed, it is necessary** to start being engaged according to the given chapter "6 Part two of the universal method of drugless treatment for depression, chronic fatigue syndrome, other neurological diseases and hypertension" and to do it 1-2 weeks, then, it is necessary to be engaged 1-2 weeks according to the chapter "3 Part one of the universal method of drugless treatment for depression, chronic fatigue syndrome, other neurological diseases and hypertension" of the present book again, then again, it is necessary to be engaged according to the present chapter "6 Part two of the universal method of drugless treatment for depression, chronic fatigue syndrome, other neurological diseases and hypertension" 1-2 weeks, etc.

I would like to repeat important advice: It is not recommended to drink even light alcoholic drinks. Some undesirable reaction, besides, rejecting back on several parameters, takes place.

7 The text of the author of the method pronounced by him in a demonstration video

Good day. I am the author of the "Methods of active self-regulation for deliverance from depression…" *(it is part of working title of the suggested method)*. This method is based on the inevident, latent mechanisms of influence on a human organism. Now, I will show you, so to say, external actions at occupation by the methods. There are also several, so to speak, internal moments. It is told about them in detail in the text of the Part one *("3 Part one of the universal method of drugless treatment for depression, chronic fatigue syndrome, other neurological diseases and hypertension")* of the method. It should be mentioned that it is not necessary to pronounce phrases as loudly as I do. Whisper is enough. Pay attention to hysterical intonation at pronouncing the phrases. This moment is important. So:

1. Yes, I shouldn't die, yes, I will live forever *(these phrases are repeatedly pronounced by the author during approximately a minute and he does necessary movements thus)*.
2. Yes, I take pleasure *(this phrase is repeatedly pronounced by the author during approximately a minute and he does necessary movements thus)*.
3. Yes, I recover *(this phrase is repeatedly pronounced by the author during approximately a minute and he does necessary movements thus)*.

Then, the author repeated once again three listed above points. At moderately severe disease, these actions and phrases should be repeated in succession during fifteen-twenty minutes a day till absolute recovery.

At moderately severe depression, it is necessary to be engaged in the Part one *("3 Part one of the universal method of drugless treatment for depression, chronic fatigue syndrome, other neurological diseases and hypertension")* or Part two *("6 Part two of the universal method of drugless treatment for depression, chronic fatigue syndrome, other neurological diseases and hypertension")* of the methods fifteen-twenty minutes. You can do feet bath *(salt bath for the feet)* simultaneously, however, it is not obligingly. For the feet bath *(salt bath for the feet)*, use a basin with warm water with the salt dissolved in it as it is described in a chapter "Feet bath" *("5 Feet bath")* of the given method.

8 Notes

It should be mentioned once again that, besides the author, only one person from those, whom the method was tested on, did feet bath (salt bath for the feet). Following advice of the author should be mentioned too: If you do feet bath (salt bath for the feet) not in a context of occupation by Sahaja yoga but in the context of occupation according to the chapters **"3 Part one of the universal method of drugless treatment for depression, chronic fatigue syndrome, other neurological diseases and hypertension"** and **"6 Part two of the universal method of drugless treatment for depression, chronic fatigue syndrome, other neurological diseases and hypertension"** of the present book, it is not necessary to do feet bath (salt bath for the feet) more than half a year, while, it is possible to be engaged according to the mentioned chapters **"3 Part one of the universal method of drugless treatment for depression, chronic fatigue syndrome, other neurological diseases and hypertension"** and **"6 Part two of the universal method of drugless treatment for depression, chronic fatigue syndrome, other neurological diseases and hypertension"** of the present book (but already without doing feet baths (salt baths for the feet)) beyond all bounds for a long time.

At a choice of degree of vigor of performance of the movements accompanying pronouncing the phrases, be guided by your own sensations of comfort. It is appropriate here to adduce once again advice from the chapters **"3 Part one of the universal method of drugless treatment for depression, chronic fatigue syndrome, other neurological diseases and hypertension"** and **"6 Part two of the universal method of drugless treatment for depression, chronic fatigue syndrome, other neurological diseases and hypertension"** of the present book: Choice of the moment of transition from one pose and/or type of movements and/or phrase to other pose and/or type of movements and/or phrase should be done guiding by condition of disappearance of feeling of comfort at carrying out any certain pose and/or type of movements and/or phrase that is a signal to its/their change.

9 About the method

Local testing of the method is finished successfully. Results are positive.

The citation from a book [15]:

"Depression harms to health more than such chronic diseases as stenocardia, arthritis, asthma and diabetes. Scientists from World Health Organization (WHO) have reported about it. Worst condition is at those diseased ones whose depression is combined with any chronic illness.

Doctor Somnat Chatterji together with colleagues from WHO surveyed more than 240 thousand persons in 60 countries of the world and has come to a conclusion that depression influences a state of health in much greater degrees than other illnesses do, reports Reuters.

During research, it was found out that on the average from 9 % to 23 % of people in addition to asthma, stenocardia, arthritis and/or diabetes had depression signs. Scientists have found out that the worst combination is depression and diabetes. "If you are sick of diabetes and depression throughout a year your possibilities are reduced to 40 %", - doctor Chatterji considers.

As a whole, research has shown necessity of more attentive relation to depression treatment. "We try to prove that if sick people are subject to influence of depression (in addition to the main illness) and the doctor doesn't try to treat it condition of the person won't improve despite treatment for the main illness, since depression will worsen condition of the patient each time", - has noted Chatterji. Besides, scientists urge doctors to check, at diagnosing, patients on presence of signs of depression."

The given method was created exclusively with intention to help to people suffering from depression, however, it proved to be enough universal owing to universality of therapeutic effect of the method, about which in more detail:

The therapeutic effect of the "Method of magic phrases and movements" (it is part of former (working) title of the present method) is based on three powerful know-hows. The main know-how is so inevident and, at the same time, so true that if the author of this method would not exist, unfortunately, mankind it's unlikely would receive it at its disposal. In other words, the method is penetrated through and through by such logic, which it is very difficult, even it is simply impossible, to guess to, and by some of thousand-year knowledge in the field of esoterics, which also it was necessary to guess to choose from its (of knowledge) long line and to use for the aims of the method. However, in the method, there is no used knowledge from esoterics in the pure state. This knowledge has only impulsed for creation of some (minor) know-hows (secrets). While, the main know-how (secret) entirely belongs to the author. The author explains the fact of creation of this method so that, in fact, he has reached the last, the eighth stage of yoga, which the true opens from, and it allowed him to create this method, which secrets it is very difficult to guess to for usual person.

Indications to application:

- Depression conditions;
- Chronic fatigue syndrome, sharp decrease of capacity for work, undue fatigability;
- Other neurological diseases;
- Hypertension;
- High frequency of stressful situations;
- Any chronic diseases;
- Memory impairment;
- Deterioration of mutual relations with an inner circle.

Expected effect:

- Exit from depression;
- Exit from condition of chronic fatigue syndrome, decrease of capacity for work, undue fatigability;
- Recovery from other neurological diseases;
- Pressure normalization;
- Self-appraisal and self-esteem rising;
- Improvement of health and mutual relations with the inner circle;
- More successful any purposeful activity with smaller metabolic cost;
- Fast restoration of capacity for work after (and during) stresses, illnesses, serious physical and mental loads;
- Decrease of uneasiness and deliverance from baseless scares.

According to the author of the given method, even each healthy person, for effective prophylaxis and counteraction to negative influence of aggressive information medium, should be engaged in the present method every year two weeks, which are apart for approximately half a year or exactly half a year for ten-fifteen minutes a day. In other words, the method renders very favorable effect as prophylaxis.

Citations from a case history of one of the tested ones are as follows:

"This man sick of depression and simultaneously of chronic fatigue syndrome is ill about four years and it was far not the first such episode of this illness. For achievement of stable effect of condition improvement, one and a half month of occupation by the given method for twenty minutes a day was required to the patient. After that, he was engaged approximately two months else fifteen minutes a day.

By the current moment, aforementioned person sick of depression is not engaged in the method already more than six years. However, his condition stabilized and, moreover, any traces of depression did not remain."

The importance of the method:

Depression and chronic fatigue syndrome are enough widespread illnesses. By data of World Health Organization (WHO), about 20-30 % of the population of the globe suffer from periodically becoming aggravated depression. And this number constantly grows, although, actually nobody knows the real digit. This results from the fact that it is impossible to carry out general checkup of all population of the globe.

Depression is considered as one of the most excruciating and hard to cure diseases. There is even an opinion that the one who will find a way of treatment for depression deserves the Nobel Prize. As to present method, it can't be nominated for the Nobel Prize, since it is not science-intensive. It is possible to put down this to its advantages, since there are not any side effects from the method.

Efficiency of the method at hypertension:

Among cured ones, there is also a woman who suffered from hypertension. The top pressure indication 180 and 200 was not rare for her. Even those preparations, which have been prescribed to her in several hospitals, which she laid for the last years in, did not help. The given method helped in two weeks of occupation according to its chapter **"3 Part one of the universal method of drugless treatment for depression, chronic fatigue syndrome, other neurological diseases and hypertension"** for ten minutes a day in position sitting on a chair or armchair. Now, pressure doesn't exceed norm.

Rejuvenating effect and treatment for other diseases:

It is noticed that some dilution of faeces, which start to remind infantile ones slightly that speaks about rejuvenating effect, is observed at all those engaged in the method. Therefore, most probably, the given method is capable to help to those ones suffering from constipations too. Supposition of the author that many other diseases can be cured too is based in considerable degree on that the offered method treats thanks just to the general rejuvenation of the organism.

Degree of complexity of the method:

You can pay attention to that, as a matter of fact, the described method comes to carrying out several simple movements, to pronouncing several phrases and to concentration on sense of phrases, on the vertical from the brain to the tailbone, which area endocrine glands are located in, to concentration on the brain and on the trunk. An important point is the accurate synchronism of carrying out movements and pronouncing phrases.

Degree of novelty and safety of the method:

Creation of the given method reminds known history of the invention of Galileo Galilei - a telescope. Galilei has guessed to bridge two lenses and a pipe in a single whole. The present method also successfully unites knowledge from different areas. And, despite it, the method differs by very big and basic novelty. Full safety of the method is obvious as well.

Influence of the method on endocrine system:

Described in the present method mechanism completely excluding introduction of chemical substances in the organism from the outside very effectively stimulates development in the organism of own endorphins at the expense of active stimulation of endocrine glands based on having accurate logic substantiation know-how (secret) allowing to influence on a part of endocrine system or even on entire endocrine system. Combination of such two aspects as meditative immersion and activation of endocrine system gives striking by efficiency result.

10 Testimonial of the person who was seriously sick of depression and, simultaneously, of chronic fatigue syndrome

"Hello,

When I was 34 years old, I was sick of serious depression throughout very long time (more than 3 years) and it was far not the first episode of this illness. However, this time, everything was much longer and illness degree was much greater. Who was sick of depression sometime will understand how it is when arms and feet are safe but there are not any forces even elementary to walk not to mention work, feelings, friends. It is the uttermost gulf and God only knows when this misfortune will pass. Not everyone is capable to be kept from suicide at those sensations, which I experienced. Naturally, serious medical treatment, which included both a considerable quantity of drugs and various types of physiotherapy, was done, there were even several sessions on transfusion and clearing blood (plasmapheresis). However, nothing helped and when duration of illness has already considerably exceeded the previous episodes, I have panicked that, probably, it will pass never. Doctors couldn't guarantee to me anything accurately. They reassured by words and changed drugs only. One day, I found out that there is such "Universal method of drugless treatment for depression, chronic fatigue syndrome, other neurological diseases and hypertension". I have started to be engaged in it for 20 minutes a day at first. It was very difficult to me but I had not any chances and ways to recover any more and, therefore I, was engaged and engaged through "I can't" and "I do not want". In one and a half month, I felt that forces like have started to increase somewhat and I already could go on walks near to the house. I began to be engaged in the method 15 minutes a day and, in a month, I became still better, i.e. I was let unhealthy at all but it was already possible to live somehow. One day, the moment when something has matured in me has come, some power volcano erupted outside and I became almost good within 2 days but I haven't stopped occupations. And in two weeks, I felt as well as before illness, which excruciated me more than 3 years. I am very grateful to the author of the given method."

Bibliography

1. "Chakras." <u>Internet center "Recovery" // Your health is in your arms</u>. 2008. Internet center "Recovery", Saratov, Russia. 8 Jan. 2014. <<u>http://www.kornilov-s-a.ru/chakras/chakras-2.htm</u>>

2. "Meditation Audio and video practises." <u>Internet center "Recovery" // Your health is in your arms</u>. 2012. Internet center "Recovery", Saratov, Russia. 8 Jan. 2014. <<u>http://www.kornilov-s-a.ru/audio.htm</u>>

3. Anan'ev V.A. "Silence temple." <u>MP3 music // Archive of MP3 music</u>. 2014. 8 Jan. 2014. <<u>http://musicmp3spb.org/album/v_a_ananjev_hram_tishiny.html</u>>

4. Patrushev, Andrey. "Recovery: on the magic river." <u>Internet page for possibility to order mind machines and other devices and disks</u>. 2014. 8 Jan. 2014. <<u>http://www.mindmachine.ru/audiostrobe/patrushev/river.htm</u>>

5. Patrushev, Andrey. "Recovery: on the magic river." <u>Information and educational portal of Kuzbass and cities of Siberia</u>. 2014. 8 Jan. 2014. <<u>http://locman.hutor.ru/ebook_info/999</u>>

6. "Site about maintenance of a healthy condition of an organism by own efforts of the person." <u>Internet center "Recovery" // Your health is in your arms</u>. 2012. Internet center "Recovery", Saratov, Russia. 8 Jan. 2014. <<u>http://www.kornilov-s-a.ru/</u>>

7. "Method of opening chakras." <u>Internet center "Recovery" // Your health is in your arms</u>. 2012. Internet center "Recovery", Saratov, Russia. 8 Jan. 2014. <<u>http://www.kornilov-s-a.ru/chakras/chakras-4.htm</u>>

8. "Method of opening chakras." <u>Internet center "Recovery" // Your health is in your arms</u>. 2011. Internet center "Recovery", Saratov, Russia. 8 Jan. 2014. <<u>http://www.kornilov-s-a.ru/chakras/chakras-4-01.htm</u>>

9. "Video with demonstration of EFT Emotional Freedom Technique for insomnia." <u>Bravica</u>. 2013. Bravica Inc. Jan. 2014. <<u>http://bravica.tv/video_d1mqUPm7L5A.htm</u>>

10. "Video-sharing website." <u>Youtube</u>. 2014. Google Inc. 8 Jan. 2014. <<u>http://www.youtube.com</u>>

11. "EFT Emotional Freedom Technique INSOMNIA." <u>Youtube</u>. 2014. Google Inc. 8 Jan. 2014. <<u>http://www.youtube.com/watch?v=d1mqUPm7L5A</u>>

12. "Demonstration of the universal method of drugless treatment for depression, chronic fatigue syndrome, other neurological diseases and hypertension." <u>Youtube</u>. 2014. Google Inc. 20 Jan. 2014. <<u>http://youtu.be/CxKqD41SF9A</u>>

13. Jasmuheen. *Pranic Nourishment.* Self Empowerment Academy. Australia. 2006. Print.

14. Jasmuheen. "Pranic Nourishment // Nutrition for the new millenium." <u>E-book</u>. 2006. 20 Jan. 2014. <<u>http://www.baytallaah.com/bookspdf/142.pdf</u>>

15. Yu. Sherbatykh. "How to remain young and to live longly." <u>E-book</u>. 2014. 28 Jan. 2014. <<u>http://books.google.ru/books?id=K43GSVBJ5eAC&printsec=frontcover&hl=ru#v=onepage&q&f=false</u>>

Printed in the United States
By Bookmasters